# Medical Management of
# Pregnancy Complicated by Diabetes

## FIFTH EDITION

Edited by
**Donald R. Coustan, MD**

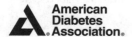
American Diabetes Association.

*Director, Book Publishing*, Abe Ogden; *Managing Editor*, Greg Guthrie; *Acquisitions Editor*, Victor Van Beuren; *Editorial Services*, Cenveo Publisher Services; *Production Manager*, Melissa Sprott; *Composition*, ADA; *Cover Design*, Jody Billert; *Printer*, United Graphics.

Printed in the United States of America
1 3 5 7 9 10 8 6 4 2

The suggestions and information contained in this publication are generally consistent with the *Clinical Practice Recommendations* and other policies of the American Diabetes Association, but they do not represent the policy or position of the Association or any of its boards or committees. Reasonable steps have been taken to ensure the accuracy of the information presented. However, the American Diabetes Association cannot ensure the safety or efficacy of any product or service described in this publication. Individuals are advised to consult a physician or other appropriate health-care professional before undertaking any diet or exercise program or taking any medication referred to in this publication. Professionals must use and apply their own professional judgment, experience, and training and should not rely solely on the information contained in this publication before prescribing any diet, exercise, or medication. The American Diabetes Association—its officers, directors, employees, volunteers, and members—assumes no responsibility or liability for personal or other injury, loss, or damage that may result from the suggestions or information in this publication.

♾ The paper in this publication meets the requirements of the ANSI Standard Z39.48-1992 (permanence of paper).

ADA titles may be purchased for business or promotional use or for special sales. To purchase more than 50 copies of this book at a discount, or for custom editions of this book with your logo, contact the American Diabetes Association at the address below, at booksales@diabetes.org, or by calling 703-299-2046.

American Diabetes Association
1701 North Beauregard Street
Alexandria, Virginia 22311

DOI: 10.2337/9781580405102

**Library of Congress Cataloging-in-Publication Data**
Medical management of pregnancy complicated by diabetes / Donald R. Coustan, editor. -- 5th ed.
p. ; cm.
Includes bibliographical references and index.
ISBN 978-1-58040-510-2 (alk. paper)
I. Coustan, Donald R. II. American Diabetes Association.
[DNLM: 1. Pregnancy in Diabetics--therapy. 2. Diabetes Mellitus. 3. Diabetes, Gestational--therapy. 4. Pregnancy Outcome. WQ 248]
618.3--dc23
                    2012049594

*This book is dedicated to the many mothers with diabetes
who have allowed us to participate in their care over the years,
being involved in the most important events in their families' lives.
We continue to learn from each of you,
and applying those lessons has advanced our ability
to care for women with diabetes during their pregnancies.*

# Contents

Nutrition Management of Preexisting Diabetes During Pregnancy   75

# Foreword

This fifth edition is intended to provide up-to-date guidance on all aspects of the care of pregnant women with preexisting diabetes, whether she has type 1 or type 2 diabetes, and with gestational diabetes. The care of pregnant women with diabetes and gestational diabetes requires a committed health-care team and considerable resources. It is our hope that the information in this book will be helpful in enabling the various health-care professionals who make up that team to have access to practical advice and carry out their mission. Each of the contributors is engaged actively in providing care to pregnant women with preexisting diabetes and gestational diabetes. Although there are many reasonable approaches to providing that care, we have outlined herein those that we find to be effective.

# Acknowledgments

The editor is indebted to Dr. Lois Jovanovič, who lovingly edited the first four editions of this book. She has set a high standard for this fifth edition. Her contributions to our understanding of diabetes in pregnancy and its treatment have been seminal.

In addition to the contributors to this current fifth edition, the editor would like to acknowledge the important contributions of the many health professionals who have contributed to previous editions of this book; the current edition is built on a very strong foundation:

Richard M. Cowett, MD

Stephanie Dunbar, MPH, RD

Donna Jornsay, RN, BSN, CPNP, MSS, ACSW

Sue Kirkman, MD

John L. Kitzmiller, MD

Lisa Marasco, MA, IBCLC, FILCA

Noreen Hall Papatheodorou, MSS, ACSW

Anne M. Patterson, RD, MPH

# List of Contributors

**EDITOR-IN-CHIEF**
**Donald R. Coustan**, MD
Maternal-Fetal Medicine Specialist
Women & Infants Hospital of
   Rhode Island
Providence, RI
Professor of Obstetrics and
   Gynecology
Warren Alpert Medical School of
   Brown University
Providence, RI

**Susan Biastre**, RD, LDN, CDE
Clinical Nutrition Specialist
Women & Infants Hospital of
   Rhode Island
Providence, RI

**Julie M. Daley**, RN, MS, CDE
Teaching Associate in Obstetrics and
   Gynecology
Warren Alpert Medical School of
   Brown University
Senior Diabetes Nurse Clinician
Division of Maternal-Fetal Medicine
Women & Infants Hospital of
   Rhode Island
Providence, RI

**Carol J. Homko**, RN, PhD, CDE
Associate Research Professor,
Departments of Medicine
(Section of Endocrinology) and
   Obstetrics & Gynecology
Temple University School of Medicine
Philadelphia, PA

**Siri Kjos**, MD, MSEd
Professor
Department of Obstetrics and
   Gynecology
Harbor UCLA Medical Center
Torrance, CA

**Abbot R. Laptook**, MD
Medical Director, Neonatal Intensive
   Care Unit
Women & Infants Hospital of
   Rhode Island
Providence, RI
Professor of Pediatrics
Warren Alpert Medical School of
   Brown University
Providence, RI

# Prepregnancy Counseling, Assessment, and Management of Women with Preexisting Diabetes or Previous Gestational Diabetes

# Highlights
# Prepregnancy Counseling, Assessment, and Management of Women with Preexisting Diabetes or Previous Gestational Diabetes

■ With proper counseling and management by the health-care team, the outcome of most pregnancies complicated by diabetes can approach that for the general population.

■ General guidelines for prepregnancy counseling and management of women with preexisting diabetes are as follows:

- Ensure that pregnancy is planned; counsel the woman about contraception methods.
- Clearly identify for the woman and her partner the risks of congenital anomalies and spontaneous abortions and their relation to glucose control.
- Provide realistic information about chronic complications of type 1 diabetes (T1D) and type 2 diabetes (T2D), their potential impact on pregnancy and childbearing, and the effect of pregnancy on chronic complications.
- Assess the woman's fitness for pregnancy, paying special attention to retinopathy, nephropathy, hypertension, neuropathy, and ischemic heart disease.
- Identify any gynecologic abnormalities before conception, and treat infertility as early as possible in view of the risk to pregnancy associated with increasing duration of diabetes and advancing maternal age. Social, financial, and marital factors permitting, pregnancy should not be discouraged.
- Provide genetic counseling, including the risks of advanced maternal age, if applicable.
- Provide realistic information about additional medical costs associated with a pregnancy complicated by diabetes, such as extra office visits, possible hospitalization, special tests, and possible intensive neonatal care.
- Achieve optimum control of blood glucose levels before conception. Ideally, A1C should be normal or near normal before discontinuing contraception.
- Encourage good general principles of health, nutrition, and hygiene, including cessation of smoking and alcohol consumption. Prescribe a prenatal vitamin with folate as part of the preconception treatment plan.
- Identify any problems requiring psychosocial consultation.
- Once the decision is made to attempt pregnancy, provide appropriate optimism that careful glycemic control and meticulous obstetric care results in an excellent outcome in the vast majority of patients.

- Diagnose pregnancy as early as possible and document conception date.

■ Counseling and management of women with previous gestational diabetes should include the following:
- Testing for diabetes or prediabetes, measuring glucose levels, and assessing the need for treatment if diabetes or prediabetes is found.
- Evaluating weight status and advising weight reduction if appropriate.
- Reviewing risks:
  ☐ Gestational diabetes in future pregnancy (~60–70% risk).
  ☐ T2D (~50–75% risk if woman is obese).

- Advising careful family planning with use of effective contraception until pregnancy is desired.

■ Problems remaining in the care of pregnant women with diabetes are as follows:
- Higher incidence of congenital anomalies and spontaneous abortions than in the nondiabetic population.
- The woman with severe complications of diabetes.
- The "difficult" or nonadherent patient.
- Education of health-care professionals and women with diabetes of childbearing age regarding the importance of preconception planning and care.

# Prepregnancy Counseling, Assessment and Management of Women with Preexisting Diabetes or Previous Gestational Diabetes

Women with diabetes in pregnancy are divided into two categories: *1)* those with diabetes that predates the pregnancy and *2)* those whose diabetes develops during the pregnancy, known as gestational diabetes mellitus (GDM). In both categories, when left untreated, the diabetes can significantly increase the risk of maternal and fetal or neonatal morbidity and mortality. Prepregnancy care incorporated into the plan of management for women with preexisting diabetes can result in improved pregnancy outcomes. This chapter provides the rationale behind and protocols for developing a prepregnancy program for women with diabetes or who have had previous gestational diabetes.

## PREEXISTING DIABETES

Women with preexisting diabetes (type 1 diabetes [T1D] or type 2 diabetes [T2D]) who desire pregnancy present a broad array of challenging problems for the health-care team. In the preinsulin era, maternal mortality was as high as 44%, and perinatal mortality was 60% (Hare 1977). Children with true T1D, however, seldom lived to childbearing ages. After the discovery of insulin, maternal and fetal or neonatal survival improved dramatically. During the past four decades, advances in the care of the individual with diabetes in general, as well as advances in fetal surveillance and neonatal care, have continued to improve outcomes in most diabetic pregnancies to near that of the general population (Coustan 1980, Jovanovic 1982, Steel 1994). The most common maternal (Table 1.1) and fetal or neonatal (Table 1.2) complications have decreased dramatically.

### Table 1.1 Examples of Maternal Complications in Diabetic Pregnancy

- Hypoglycemia, ketoacidosis
- Pregnancy-induced hypertension and preeclampsia
- Pyelonephritis, other infections
- Polyhydramnios
- Preterm labor
- Worsening of chronic complications—retinopathy, nephropathy, neuropathy, cardiac disease

## Table 1.2 Examples of Potential Perinatal Morbidity or Mortality in Infants of Mothers with Diabetes

- Asphyxia
- Birth injury
- Cardiac hypertrophy and heart failure
- Congenital anomalies
- Erythremia (increased red blood cells) and hyperviscosity
- Hyperbilirubinemia
- Hypocalcemia
- Hypoglycemia
- Hypomagnesemia
- Intrauterine growth restriction
- Macrosomia
- Neurological instability; irritability
- Organomegaly
- Respiratory distress syndrome
- Stillbirth

Despite the advances made in the care of the pregnant woman with diabetes, several problems remain:

- A high prevalence of congenital anomalies and spontaneous abortions (SABs) in infants of mothers with diabetes (IDMs)
- Care of the woman with severe complications of diabetes
- Care of the "difficult patient" who often presents late for antenatal care or is nonadherent (Steel 1994)

Morbidity and mortality associated with major congenital anomalies and SAB are of major concern. The magnitude of both appears to be related to metabolic control. The true prevalence of SAB pregnancies is not known, but it has been reported to be as high as 30–60%, depending on the degree of hyperglycemia at the time of conception, which is double that of the general population (Miodovnik 1984). The increased risk of congenital anomalies in IDMs ranges from 6% to 12%, a two- to fivefold increase over the 2–3% incidence observed in the general population (Kitzmiller 1978, Reece 1988). This increased risk of congenital anomalies accounts for ~40% of the perinatal loss in IDMs (Reece 1986). The combined risk of congenital anomalies and SAB in poorly controlled diabetes in early pregnancy can approach 65% (Greene 1993). In a nationwide prospective study, which included first-trimester questionnaires filled out by all pregnant women with T1D in the Netherlands over a 1-year interval, congenital malformations occurred in 4.2% of self-reported planned pregnancies but in 12.2% of unplanned pregnancies (Evers 2004). Congenital malformations also increased when the mother has T2D (Macintosh 2006).

The types of congenital anomalies observed in IDMs are varied (Table 1.3). Most are of cardiac, neural tube, or skeletal origin; they are more commonly multiple, more severe, and more often fatal than those found in the general population.

## Table 1.3 Congenital Malformations in Infants of Mothers with Diabetes

| Anomaly | Ratios of Incidence* |
|---|---|
| Caudal regression | 252 |
| Spina bifida, hydrocephalus, or other central nervous system defect | 2 |
| Anencephalus | 3 |
| Heart anomalies | 4 |
| Anal or rectal atresia | 3 |
| Renal anomalies | 5 |
| Agenesis | 6 |
| Cystic kidney | 4 |
| Ureter duplex | 23 |
| Situs inversus | 84 |

* Ratio of incidence is in comparison to the general population. Heart anomalies include transposition of the great vessels, ventricular septal defect, and atrial septal defect.

Adapted from Mills JL, Baker L, Goldman AS: Malformations in infants of diabetic mothers occur before the seventh gestational week: implications for treatment. *Diabetes* 28:292–293, 1979

The etiology of this increased prevalence of congenital anomalies in IDMs has been the subject of intense research. In an experimental setting, hyperglycemia and other metabolic abnormalities are teratogenic, singly or in combination (Kalter 1983; Freinkel 1984; Reece 1986, 1988; Sadler 1989). Fetal organogenesis is largely complete by 9 weeks after the last menstrual period (7 weeks postconception) (Mills 1979). Poorly controlled diabetes during the early weeks of pregnancy, in many cases before a woman even knows that she has conceived, significantly increases the risk of a first-trimester SAB or delivering an infant with a major anomaly (Greene 1989).

The A1C, which expresses an average of the circulating glucose for the 4–6 weeks before its measurement, has become a useful tool in assessing a woman's metabolic control early in pregnancy, during the critical period of organogenesis. Several studies have shown a definite association between A1C levels in early pregnancy (<13 weeks) and increased risk of congenital anomalies and SABs (Fig. 1.1) (Miller 1981, Ylinen 1984, Greene 1989). In one recent study, a maternal A1C of 11% in the periconceptional period was associated with a 1 in 7 (14%) risk of congenital malformations (Eidem 2010). Figure 1.1 depicts the risk of malformations associated with varying levels of A1C in early pregnancy.

| A1CSD | Corresponding A1C (%)* | Absolute risk of a congenital anomaly (%, 95% confidence interval) |
|---|---|---|
| 0 | 5.5 | 2.2 (0.0–4.4) |
| 1 | 6.2 | 2.7 (0.2–5.2) |
| 2 | 6.9 | 3.2 (0.4–6.1) |
| 3 | 7.6 | 3.9 (0.7–7.2) |
| 4 | 8.3 | 4.8 (1.0–8.6) |
| 5 | 9.0 | 5.8 (1.3–10.2) |
| 6 | 9.7 | 7.0 (1.7–12.3) |
| 7 | 10.4 | 8.4 (2.0–14.8) |
| 8 | 11.1 | 10.1 (2.3–17.8) |
| 9 | 11.8 | 12.1 (2.6–21.5) |
| 10 | 12.5 | 14.4 (2.8–25.9) |
| 11 | 13.2 | 17.0 (2.9–31.1) |
| ≥ 12** | ≥13.9 | 20.1 (3.0–37.1) |

*Assumes a mean (SD) A1C assay reference value of 5.5% (0.7%) among nondiabetic, nonpregnant control subjects.
**Values of A1C standard deviation >12 were truncated to a value of 12 in the analysis.
Guerin A, Nisenbaum R, Ray JG. Use of maternal GHb concentration to estimate the risk of congenital anomalies in the offspring of women with prepregnancy diabetes. *Diabetes Care* 30:1920–1925, 2007 [online appendix 2]

**Figure 1.1** Derived Absolute Risk of a Major or Minor Congenital Anomaly in Association with the Number of Standard Deviations of Glycosylated Hemoglobin (A1C) above Normal, and the Approximate Corresponding A1C Concentration, Measured Periconceptionally

As a result of these findings, high-risk perinatal centers have developed programs for preconceptional management of the woman with diabetes who is planning a pregnancy. Women are evaluated and counseled about the risks of pregnancy, with particular emphasis on the importance of normalizing blood glucose levels periconceptionally to reduce the risks of delivering an infant with a major birth defect. Studies from these centers have confirmed that normalizing blood glucose levels before and during the early weeks of pregnancy can reduce the risk of development of major anomalies, as well as the occurrence of SAB in IDMs, to near that of the nondiabetic population (Führmann 1984, Johnstone 1990, Kitzmiller 1991). A meta-analysis concluded that preconception care can reduce the rate of anomalies by 75% (Wahabi 2010). Thus, prepregnancy counseling and management have emerged as vital components in the care of the woman with diabetes (Steel 1985). The goals of such a program are listed in Table 1.4. A practical method for organizing and implementing a program for preconception care is outlined in this chapter. Major topics include prepregnancy counseling, assessment, and management.

## Table 1.4 Goals of Prepregnancy Planning Program

- Assessment of a woman's fitness for pregnancy
- Obstetric evaluation
- Intensive education of woman and family
- Attainment of optimum diabetic control
- Timing and planning of pregnancy

## PREPREGNANCY COUNSELING

Prepregnancy counseling for the woman with diabetes ideally should begin at the onset of puberty and continue until permanent sterilization or menopause, thus encompassing all women with diabetes of childbearing potential. Furthermore, these women should be divided into two categories—those planning a pregnancy within the near future and those wanting to delay pregnancy. For women not currently planning a pregnancy, general information can be given regarding the risks of pregnancy and the importance of appropriate birth control and prepregnancy planning. Even the teenage girl who may not be thinking in terms of pregnancy needs to be questioned regarding her menstrual history and sexual activity. Her physician should provide her with information about the importance of planning one's family in the future.

For the woman contemplating pregnancy soon, a preconception consultation is essential. The major components of preconception counseling include the following:

- Contraceptive advice
- Risks of pregnancy, maternal and fetal and neonatal
- Importance of maintaining normal blood glucose levels
- Genetic counseling
- Personal commitment by the woman and her family

A preconception visit is the ideal time to introduce the woman with diabetes to the concept of a health-care team, assembled to provide the best possible care for diabetic pregnancy. The team consists of physicians, nurses and other health-care providers, dietitians, and social workers, all with expertise in this area. The physicians on the team may include a specialist in maternal-fetal medicine or obstetrics, with special expertise and interest in diabetic pregnancy and a diabetologist or internist, with special interest in pregnancy. In some centers, one physician fills both of these roles, whereas in other centers, individuals come together to form the team. Other specialists often are included as needed—for example, a nephrologist or ophthalmologist may play a major role when the patient with diabetes has vascular complications. Diabetes nurse educators generally have the greatest amount of contact with the patient, touching base frequently to help with the maintenance of good metabolic control. A neonatologist or pediatrician is also an important member of the team, providing information to the patient regarding what to expect after the baby is born.

A planned pregnancy is a major objective of preconception counseling; thus, establishing an effective contraceptive method must be an early priority in pre-pregnancy planning (see also chapter 2). The health-care provider should review with the woman her options for contraception and help her choose the one most appropriate for her situation.

The health-care provider should explain to the woman the risks of pregnancy to her developing baby (Table 1.2) as well as to herself (Table 1.1) (see also chapter 10). This prepregnancy counseling session is the ideal moment to emphasize to the woman her two- to fivefold increased risk of having a baby with a congenital anomaly and her increased risk for having a first-trimester SAB if blood glucose levels are not well controlled. This is the crucial time to underscore these particular problems so that the patient will understand fully the rationale behind precon-ception care with the effort toward normalizing blood glucose levels before and during the early weeks of pregnancy. She should be apprised that organogenesis is largely complete by the ninth week of gestation after her last menstrual period (7th week after conception) and that, with efforts to normalize blood glucose lev-els, her risk for having a baby with a congenital anomaly or an early SAB can be reduced significantly (Fig. 1.1). Furthermore, she can be assured that with contin-ued optimal glucose control throughout pregnancy, she can effectively reduce her risk of developing further complications.

The health-care provider should advise the woman of her own personal risks when undertaking pregnancy, emphasizing to her the need for evaluation for the presence of diabetic complications and other general medical problems before conception. She will need to know that the chronic complications of diabetes can worsen during pregnancy, although debate persists as to whether the pregnancy itself influences the natural course of these complications. Certainly, retinopathy has been known to progress in some patients during pregnancy (Phelps 1986, Elman 1990, Chew 1995, Henricsson 1999, Diabetes Control and Complications Trial Research Group 2000, Sheth 2002, Loukovaara 2003). If the woman has known renal insufficiency or severe gastroenteropathy, she should be advised that these conditions constitute significant risks to both mother and developing infant and, in some individuals, may be relative contraindications to pregnancy. The presence of ischemic heart disease, known to be associated with significant maternal mortality, is in most cases a contraindication to pregnancy. Thus, pre-conception evaluation of these potential complications must be emphasized.

Although these risks are obviously serious, emphasis can be placed on the evidence accumulated to date—namely, that for most women, intensive manage-ment of the diabetes with the goal of normalizing blood glucose levels before and during the entire pregnancy can result in outcomes similar to those of the non-diabetic population.

Genetics is another important aspect of preconception counseling. The woman with diabetes may be reassured that it is rare for a newborn to develop diabetes. If she has T1D and is ≥25 years old, the chance of her child developing T1D at some point is ~1%; if she is <25 years old, this chance increases to ~4% (Warram 1991). If both parents have T1D, the risk is higher, in the range of 10–25% (Warram 1991). T2D is present in ~11% of the adult U.S. population (http://www.cdc.gov/nchs/fastats/diabetes.htm). The risk for offspring of women with T2D to eventually develop T2D ranges from 1 in 7 (14%) when the parent has developed T2D before the age of 50 years, to 1 in 13 (7.6%) when the onset was later (American Diabetes Association 2012a). Although these risks of developing diabetes are higher than that of the general population, they are not significant enough to advise a woman against pregnancy on genetic grounds.

Finally, the health-care provider must convey to each woman the importance of the deep personal commitment that she will be undertaking during the pregnancy. The demands of maintaining a routine to normalize the blood glucose are many. For some patients, the actual cost of such an undertaking may be prohibitive. The woman needs to understand that once pregnant, she will be seen frequently by her health-care team, perhaps as often as weekly. She may require hospitalization if problems with the pregnancy develop or her metabolic control deteriorates. She will be undergoing various special tests throughout the pregnancy to assess the well-being of her developing baby. She may want to check with her insurance company to see what coverage her policy offers with regard to pregnancy. Many states offer supplemental aid programs to indigent women during pregnancy. The patient can seek help through her local health department or her state's maternal or child health division.

In addition, the physician also may want to have the woman undergo psychosocial evaluation and counseling. The counselor can assist her in coping with the specific problems pertaining to pregnancy and other pressing commitments, such as small children in the family, job responsibilities, and financial burdens. If, after discussing in depth these various aspects of diabetes and pregnancy and the commitment required, the woman decides that she would like to pursue a pregnancy, she can then be scheduled for prepregnancy assessment.

## PREPREGNANCY ASSESSMENT

The prepregnancy assessment (American Diabetes Association 2004) of a woman with diabetes (Table 1.5) should begin with a detailed diabetic history, including the following:

- Type of diabetes
- Age of onset, duration, and course of disease
- Past history, including hospitalizations for treatment of acute and chronic complications
- Current diabetic regimen, with attention to routine insulin dosages, prior or current use of oral glucose-lowering agents, medical nutrition therapy and individualized meal plan, exercise, hypoglycemia unawareness, and self-monitoring of blood glucose
- History of other medical problems, especially hypertension and thyroid disease
- A careful obstetric history, with attention to contraceptive use and past history of infertility or pregnancy complications, such as pregnancy-induced hypertension, polyhydramnios, and preterm labor
- All medications that the woman is taking
- A support system, including family and work environment

## Table 1.5 Prepregnancy Assessment for Women with Diabetes

- History and physical examination
- Gynecologic evaluation
- Laboratory evaluation
  - A1C level
  - Urinalysis and culture
  - 24-h urine for creatinine clearance and total protein
  - Thyroid studies (including thyroid-stimulating hormone [TSH] level) and other testing as indicated
- Special studies
  - Electrocardiogram or treadmill
  - Neuropathy testing if indicated

The health-care provider should perform a careful physical examination with special attention not only to diabetes-related complications, but also to other organ-system abnormalities, especially hypertension. Known hypertension in a woman with diabetes should be treated promptly with medications not known to be teratogenic, such as methyldopa and hydralazine. Angiotensin-converting enzyme (ACE) inhibitors and angiotensin receptor blockers (ARBs) are contraindicated in pregnancy because of their possible teratogenicity and their known association with fetal and neonatal renal failure.

The following are recommendations concerning blood pressure control in pregnancy (Peterson 1992; Lazarus 1997; Hansson 1998; UK Prospective Diabetes Study Group 1998; Bakris 2000; Von Dadelszen 2000; Arauz-Pacheco 2002; Ochsenbein-Kolble 2004; American Diabetes Association 2005, 2012b; American College of Obstetricians and Gynecologists [ACOG] 2012):

- Nonpregnant patients with diabetes who have hypertension should be treated to a blood pressure <130 mmHg systolic and <80 mmHg diastolic.
- Pregnant women with diabetes who have chronic hypertension should receive drug therapy when lifestyle and behavioral therapy are not adequate to control blood pressure. The blood pressure level at which pharmacologic therapy should be introduced is controversial, and ranges from 140–150 mmHg systolic and from 90–100 mmHg diastolic (ACOG 2012).
- Drugs safe for pregnancy should be added sequentially until target blood pressure levels are achieved.
- ACE inhibitors and ARBs are contraindicated in pregnancy.
- Atenolol may be associated with a greater risk of small-for-gestational-age infants and should be avoided.
- Women not achieving target blood pressure despite multiple drug therapy should be referred to a physician experienced in the care of pregnant women with diabetes who have hypertension.
- All women with diabetes, especially those with hypertension, should be monitored closely for the development of preeclampsia.
- 24-h ambulatory blood pressure monitoring or blood pressure self-measurements may provide a more complete picture of the blood pressure bur-

den than isolated office blood pressure and should be considered when determining the need for or monitoring the effect of antihypertensive therapy.

The woman's eye examination should be performed through dilated pupils by an ophthalmologist. If this examination reveals preproliferative retinopathy or macular edema, proper treatment, including laser photocoagulation, should be performed and the woman's retinal status stabilized before pregnancy. Risk factors for progression of retinopathy include the following:

- Duration of diabetes
- Retinal status
- Elevated A1C
- Rapid normalization of glucose control
- Hypertension
- Valsalva maneuver (increases risk of retinal hemorrhage)

Likewise, a careful evaluation of the patient's renal status and efforts to detect the presence of autonomic and peripheral neuropathies are important.

The possible presence of cardiac disease should be evaluated carefully. If a woman has had diabetes for >10 years, or any duration of diabetes and hypertension, the health-care provider should consider obtaining an electrocardiogram and perhaps even proceed with more in-depth cardiac testing to rule out underlying ischemic heart disease, especially if the woman gives a history of chest pain.

The woman also should have a neurological assessment and lower-extremity examination for evidence of vascular disease, neuropathy, deformity, or infection (American Diabetes Association 2004).

In addition to this thorough medical assessment, the woman should undergo a careful gynecologic examination. Prompt detection and treatment of gynecologic abnormalities, such as infection or structural deformities, are advantageous. Additionally, it is important to determine from the history whether the woman has any degree of infertility, so that a specific problem can be treated early to minimize any delay for the planned pregnancy.

As part of the woman's total evaluation, the health-care provider should order the following specific baseline laboratory studies in addition to those relating to the woman's general medical status:

- Initial A1C level to evaluate her current degree of metabolic control
- Renal function, including a 24-h urine collection for creatinine clearance and total protein and microalbumin
- Clean-catch urinalysis with culture and sensitivity
- Thyroid testing that would include TSH level, and, if indicated, free T4, and antimicrosomal antibodies (American Diabetes Association 2004)

On completion of the preconception assessment, the patient will see her physician for a return counseling appointment. At that visit, her physician will review with her the results of her tests and discuss her fitness for pregnancy.

The discovery of certain diabetes-related complications may serve as absolute or relative contraindications for pregnancy (Table 1.6). If the woman is found to have clinically proven ischemic cardiac disease, the risks of maternal mortality are high, and the woman with this very serious complication should be counseled against undertaking pregnancy. Additionally, she should be asked to consider permanent sterilization.

---

## Table 1.6 Potential Contraindications to Pregnancy

- Ischemic heart disease
- Active proliferative retinopathy, untreated
- Renal insufficiency: creatinine clearance <50 ml/min or serum creatinine >2 mg/dl or heavy proteinuria (>2 g/24 h)
- Severe gastroenteropathy: nausea or vomiting and diarrhea

---

If the woman is found to have significant proliferative retinopathy, she should be advised to delay the pregnancy until the ophthalmologist can treat her eye disease appropriately and determine that the retinopathy has stabilized.

If she displays significant renal disease (serum creatinine >1.5 mg/dl or creatinine clearance <50 ml/min), she should be counseled about the high risk of morbidity and mortality for her infant that is associated with this particular complication (Combs 1993, Purdy 1996, Biesenbach 1999, Khoury 2002). Likewise, significant proteinuria (>300 mg/24 h), especially when accompanied by hypertension, portends a poor pregnancy outcome (Hare 1977, Combs 1993).

Women with nephropathy are at increased risk to develop hypertension and significant edema to the extent that it interrupts their lifestyle. A woman who has undergone renal transplantation may be able to undertake pregnancy safely if her medical status is otherwise stable, although the risk is still significant.

Severe gastroenteropathy should be considered a relative contraindication to pregnancy. Metabolic control and nutrition for both the woman and her developing baby are difficult to maintain with this particular complication.

In conclusion, if the woman shows no evidence of active diabetic complications or other health problems that place her at significant risk, she may be safely advised to begin plans for pregnancy. At this point, she may be entered into the prepregnancy management protocol.

---

## PREPREGNANCY MANAGEMENT

Once a woman has undergone prepregnancy counseling and assessment and her fitness for safely undertaking a pregnancy has been established, her health-care provider should outline a plan for prepregnancy management, the goal of which is to normalize the blood glucose levels before conception and to maintain euglycemia throughout the pregnancy.

Assuming that all preexisting complications of a woman's diabetes have been stabilized, she can then be introduced to the team concept of patient management. Ideally, her diabetes team should include the following:

■ Her primary care physician and endocrinologist or other physician with interest and experience in management of diabetes in pregnancy
■ Her maternal-fetal medicine specialist or obstetrician who is skilled in high-risk obstetrics
■ A nurse educator (preferably a certified diabetes educator)
■ A social worker
■ A registered dietitian
■ A pediatrician or neonatologist
■ Other specialist(s) as appropriate

In achieving preconception goals, the woman with diabetes benefits from effective application of diabetes self-management skills. Members of the management team, which includes diabetes educators and registered dietitians, may provide appropriate education based on assessment, intervention, and monitoring of a woman's response.

Before pregnancy, women with diabetes should be encouraged to adopt a healthy lifestyle, including a healthy diet, moderate to vigorous activity, and emotional well-being. Obesity is an independent risk factor for adverse pregnancy outcomes. Women with diabetes who are overweight (BMI 25–29.9) or obese (BMI ≥30) should be encouraged to lose weight. Weight loss can reduce insulin resistance in women who are overweight or obese, assisting glycemic control. Moderate weight loss and cardiovascular disease (CVD) risk reduction may be achieved by balancing caloric intake and physical activity.

The prepregnancy meal plan should meet nutrient recommendations based on the Institute of Medicine's Dietary Reference Intakes (DRIs) (Institute of Medicine Food and Nutrition Board 2006). Caloric needs for women are based on age and physical activity level.

### Table 1.7 Estimated Calories for Women to Achieve Calorie Balance at Different Activity Levels

| Age (years) | Sedentary | Moderately Active | Active |
|---|---|---|---|
| 19–25 | 2,000 | 2,200 | 2,400 |
| 26–45 | 1,800 | 2,000 | 2,200 |

Dietary Guidelines for Americans, 2010. United States Department of Agriculture, Center for Nutrition Policy and Promotion. http://www.cnpp.usda.gov/DGAs2010-PolicyDocument.htm. Accessed 5 September 2012

To achieve weight loss, a reduction in caloric intake or an increase in physical activity must occur. Carbohydrate management is a key factor in achieving glucose control and should be individualized. Carbohydrate from fruits, vegetables, whole grains, legumes, and low-fat milk are encouraged to meet nutrient recommendations. A pattern of three meals and some snacks can provide satiety, promote weight goals, and transition to the pregnancy meal plan. Additionally, women with diabetes should do the following:

- Limit saturated fat to <7% of total kcals.
- Minimize intake of trans fats.
- Limit dietary cholesterol to <200 mg/day.
- Reduce sodium intake to 2,300 mg/day.

The 2010 dietary guidelines (Dietary Guidelines for Americans 2010) recommend that all women in the periconceptional period consume 400 µg/day synthetic folic acid from fortified foods or supplements and additional amounts from a varied diet. Many women are prescribed a prenatal multivitamin mineral supplement.

Next, the woman should be placed on an intensive regimen of multiple injections in a basal-bolus fashion (Table 1.8), or an insulin pump if she is not already practicing an intensive regimen. If the woman has been treated with oral hypoglycemic agents, these should be discontinued and insulin therapy initiated.

## Table 1.8 Goals for Prepregnancy Daily Insulin Therapy

**Goals of therapy**
- A1C as close to normal as possible (<7%)
- Preprandial capillary plasma glucose 80–110 mg/dl (4.4–6.1 mmol/l)
- 2-h postprandial capillary plasma glucose <155 mg/dl (<8.6 mmol/l)

*From* American Diabetes Association, 2012b, 2004b.

Insulin is the mainstay of therapy for preexisting diabetes in pregnancy. Intensive insulin therapy with either three or four injections of insulin per day or the use of an insulin pump is necessary in most patients to achieve the near-normal blood glucose goals that are defined in Table 1.8. Both multiple daily injections (MDI) and continuous subcutaneous insulin infusion (CSII) use the concept of basal and bolus insulin replacement to mimic normal physiologic delivery of insulin during fasting and eating. Skills for intensive diabetes self-management are best learned before pregnancy, so that excellent glycemic control is achieved at the time of conception and during organogenesis. Unfortunately, this is not always possible, because many women have unplanned pregnancies. A woman's strong motivation to care for her fetus by improving her diabetes control, however, offers a window of opportunity to teach her skills that she may continue to use for the rest of her life.

Five insulin analogs are approved by the U.S. Food and Drug Administration (FDA) for use in nonpregnant patients. The rapid-acting insulins may improve patient adherence, decrease postmeal glucose excursions, and lower the risk of nocturnal hypoglycemia. Of the three rapid-acting insulins, lispro, glulisine, and aspart, lispro has been widely used in pregnancy without apparent adverse affects (Anderson 1997, Ebeling 1997, Brunelle 1998, Del Sindaco 1998, Colombel 1999, Lepore 2000, Bhattacharyya 2001, Idama 2001, Persson 2002, Garg 2003, Loukovaara 2003, Masson 2003, Wyatt 2004). Although large prospective randomized controlled clinical trials are not available, several retrospective and small prospective clinical trials support the safe use of lispro in pregnancy. Neither lispro (Jovanovic 1999) nor aspart (McCance 2008) appear to cross the placenta. Lispro does not appear to cause an increased incidence of congenital malformations, and it does not appear to cause an increased risk of progression of retinopathy. Both lispro and aspart appear to achieve lower 1- to 2-h postprandial glucoses levels in either gestational or preexisting diabetes compared with regular insulin (Anderson 1997, Ebeling 1997, Brunelle 1998, Del Sindaco 1998, Colombel 1999, Jovanovic 1999, Lepore 2000, Bhattacharyya 2001, Idama 2001, Persson 2002, Garg 2003, Loukovaara 2003, Masson 2003, Mecacci 2003, Pettitt 2003, Wyatt 2004). The FDA lists both lispro and aspart as safety category B. Data regarding the use of glargine in pregnancy are limited to case reports. Glargine, which does not appear to cross the placenta (Pollex 2010), is associated with a six- to eightfold increase in binding to the IGF receptor and mitogenic potency respectively compared with regular insulin (Kurtzhals 2000, Ciaraldi 2001). The mitogenic response of insulin relative to IGF-1 is ~1%. Thus, at physiologic concentrations, glargine may not display significant augmentation of mitogenic effects compared with regular insulin. The clinical significance of these binding and mitogenic effects is not known. Glargine is listed as category C by the FDA. Detemir insulin is listed as Category B by the FDA. There are no data on glulisine use in pregnancy, and it is listed as category C.

Basal insulin is used to approximate the fasting insulin requirements. When MDI therapy is used, intermediate-acting insulins such as NPH are used two to three times per day to provide basal coverage. NPH peaks at 4–10 h and has a duration of action of 10–16 h. Daytime and nighttime hypoglycemia is common in diabetic pregnancies (Kimmerle 1992, Bolli 1993). The relatively short peak action profile of NPH may explain the high risk of nocturnal hypoglycemia, even when taken at bedtime, in the setting of the low fasting glucose treatment goals established for pregnancy. A bedtime snack usually is needed to reduce this risk. Middle-of-the-night blood glucose levels should be checked occasionally depending on the clinical situation. The morning dose of intermediate-acting insulin should be given within 8–10 h after the bedtime dose to avoid hyperglycemia as the nighttime insulin concentration is waning. Predinner dosing of intermediate-acting insulin increases the risks of nocturnal hypoglycemia and fasting hyperglycemia but may be reasonable for some patients to simplify the regimen.

The long-acting insulin analog glargine (Lantus) provides steady serum levels over 24 h in patients who are not pregnant. It is FDA pregnancy category C (animal reproduction studies have shown an adverse effect on the fetus, and there are no adequate and well-controlled studies in humans, but potential benefits may warrant use of the drug in pregnant women despite potential risks). The long-acting analog detemir (Levemir) is now FDA pregnancy category B (animal reproduction studies have failed to demonstrate a risk to the fetus, and there are no adequate and well-controlled studies in pregnant women) after a randomized controlled trial comparing its use with NPH insulin in pregnancy (Mathiesen 2012). CSII uses a short- or rapid-acting insulin delivered by continuous infusion to deliver a small predetermined amount of insulin per hour. Steady-state basal levels of insulin are achieved. Titration of the basal insulin dose is based on the premeal glucose value.

Bolus insulin treatment requires an understanding of medical nutrition therapy. Rapid-acting insulin is given when carbohydrate is ingested. Rapid-acting insulin may be given with a set meal plan that involves consistent carbohydrate at meals and snacks or based on a predetermined insulin-to-carbohydrate ratio allowing for more flexible carbohydrate intake. A correction dose based on a calculated sensitivity factor is given to treat an elevated glucose value. Titration of the bolus insulin level is based on the trends of the postprandial glucose value. This approach to bolus insulin is used with both MDI and CSII.

CSII offers multiple programmable basal rates that can be especially useful for patients with nocturnal hypoglycemia and a prominent dawn phenomenon. The disadvantage of CSII is the potential for marked hyperglycemia and diabetic ketoacidosis as a consequence of insulin delivery failure. This can occur when technical problems arise with the pump, the catheter kinks, an air bubble in the tubing displaces insulin, or accidental displacement occurs at the infusion site. Women who use CSII in pregnancy can take steps to avoid the serious problem of diabetic ketoacidosis by testing blood glucose levels before and after meals, at bedtime, and within 2 h of changing the infusion set. Patients always should test blood glucose levels and ketones if symptoms of hyperglycemia and especially nausea develop, although these symptoms can be masked by pregnancy symptoms. Blood glucose levels >180 mg/dl in the absence of urine ketones should be rechecked within 2 h of a high bolus to ensure that glucose levels are improving. Glucose levels >180 mg/dl in the presence of urine ketones should be treated immediately with a subcutaneous injection. Blood glucose levels and urine ketones should be checked hourly. The infusion setup should be changed and glucose levels carefully reevaluated.

Additionally, instruction in an appropriate exercise routine will enhance the woman's physical fitness and act as an adjunct in maintaining optimal blood glucose control. Exercise is also an excellent stress reliever. Elicit the woman's psychosocial concerns, including family, job, and financial stressors, and her coping mechanisms for stress.

If the woman is not familiar with techniques for self-monitoring of blood glucose, these should be taught or reviewed (see chapter 4). She should begin testing her blood glucose levels frequently—before meals and 1 or 2 h after meals—to assess the adequacy of her insulin regimen. Preconception goals for premeal capillary glucose levels should be from 80 to 110 mg/dl (from 4.4 to 6.1 mmol/l), and 2-h postmeal glucose levels should fall below 155 mg/dl (<8.6 mmol/l) (American Diabetes Association 2004). Based on the record of a woman's self-monitoring of blood glucose, the diabetes team can then prescribe adjustments in diet, insulin, or exercise that will aid her in achieving euglycemia. If the woman is adept and well motivated, she can learn to make adjustments in her routine at home (Jovanovic 1980, American Diabetes Association 2000).

Inherent in diabetic regimens aimed at normalizing blood glucose levels is the very real risk of severe hypoglycemia (Hansson 1998). Before undertaking such a regimen, the woman and her partner should be warned about the risks of hypoglycemia. The diabetes educator should remind them about the signs, symptoms, and management of hypoglycemia, and the partner or a relative should be instructed in the use of glucagon. Proper education about hypoglycemia will result in fewer hospitalizations for this potentially life-threatening complication.

Serial A1C levels can be drawn monthly to confirm normalization of blood glucose levels in the preconception period. Normal or near-normal A1C levels (<7.0%) affirm for a woman the safety of pursuing pregnancy from a metabolic standpoint (Jovanovic 1980, 1981; American Diabetes Association 2000).

Finally, the woman should put into practice general principles of good health that may include cessation of smoking, alcohol intake, or unnecessary drugs and medications.

In addition, women with T1D are at higher risk for thyroid disorder and should have their thyroid function measured. The American Thyroid Association recommends that all women be screened for hypothyroidism during the childbearing years and that the normal range for thyroid function preconceptionally and throughout pregnancy is a free T4 of 1.0–1.6 mg/dl and a TSH in the range of 1.3–2.5 µU/l (Jovanovic 1988, American Thyroid Association 2005).

Although congenital anomalies and SABs are significantly increased in the offspring of a woman with preexisting diabetes, efforts to normalize blood glucose and A1C levels in the preconceptional period have resulted in a significant decrease in the incidence of these problems. Thus, any woman contemplating pregnancy will want to optimize her chances for a good outcome by enrolling in a preconception program that includes proper counseling, assessment, and management as outlined thus far.

## PREVIOUS GDM

A woman who has had GDM in a previous pregnancy is at significant risk to develop the following:

- GDM in subsequent pregnancies
- Type 2 diabetes in the future

For these reasons, it is important to provide the woman with a past history of GDM with information about these associated risks. Ideally, "prepregnancy" counseling should begin in the immediate postpartum period, when a woman is still sensitive to the rigors of diabetes management.

After appropriate postpartum testing, the woman should return for a counseling session with her physician, at which time the results of her postpartum glucose tests can be reviewed with her. The health-care provider should question her regarding her future pregnancy plans. During this visit, the provider can review the advantages and disadvantages of each method of birth control as it applies to her individual situation.

The provider can explain to the woman that she has an ~60–70% chance of developing GDM in future pregnancies (Philipson 1989). There is some suggestion that weight reduction before a future pregnancy may reduce the risk of recurrent GDM; thus, if obese, the woman should be strongly encouraged to lose weight before undertaking another pregnancy (American Diabetes Association 2000). During this "teachable" period, when she has just experienced the daily commitment required of a person with diabetes, she may be more motivated to follow a weight-reduction plan. If she is willing, she can be referred for effective dietary counseling.

Finally, the woman should be encouraged to have a yearly follow-up with her health-care provider. At this session, the provider can determine a fasting glucose level (normal value <100 mg/dl [<5.6 mmol/l]), assess success in weight reduction if appropriate, and review pregnancy plans. If there is any suspicion that diabetes has developed in the interim, the patient should be tested appropriately. Subsequent planning for pregnancy will depend on the findings during these annual visits. Of course, if the patient has developed diabetes and desires pregnancy, she should be enrolled immediately in the prepregnancy program described for women with preexisting diabetes (American Diabetes Association 2004).

## REFERENCES

American College of Obstetricians and Gynecologists. ACOG: Chronic hypertension in pregnancy. Practice Bulletin No. 125. American College of Obstetricians and Gynecologists. *Obstet Gynecol* 119:396–407, 2012

American Diabetes Association: Genetics of diabetes. http://www.diabetes.org/diabetes-basics/genetics-of-diabetes.html. Accessed 7 July 2012a

American Diabetes Association: Standards of medical care in diabetes—2011. *Diabetes Care* 35 (Suppl. 1):S11–S63, 2012b

American Diabetes Association: Hypertension management in adults with diabetes. *Diabetes Care* 27 (Suppl. 1):S65–S67, 2004a

American Diabetes Association: Position statement: preconception care of women with diabetes. *Diabetes Care* 27 (Suppl. 1):S76–S78, 2004b

American Diabetes Association: Nutrition recommendations and principles for people with diabetes mellitus (Position Statement). *Diabetes Care* 23 (Suppl. 1):S43–S46, 2000

American Thyroid Association: Consensus Statement #2: American Thyroid Association statement on early maternal thyroidal insufficiency: recognition, clinical management and research directions. *Thyroid* 15:77–79, 2005

Anderson JH Jr, Brunelle RL, Koivisto VA, Pfützner A, Trautmann ME, Vignati L, DiMarchi R: Reduction of postprandial hyperglycemia and frequency of hypoglycemia in IDDM patients on insulin-analog treatment: Multicenter Insulin Lispro Study Group. *Diabetes* 46:265–270, 1997

Arauz-Pacheco C, Parrott MA, Raskin P: The treatment of hypertension in patients with diabetes (Technical Review). *Diabetes Care* 25:134–147, 2002

Bakris GL, Williams M, Dworkin L, Elliott WJ, Epstein M, Toto R, Tuttle K, Douglas J, Hsueh W, Sowers J, for the National Kidney Foundation Hypertension and Diabetes Executive Committees Working Group: Preserving renal function in adults with hypertension and diabetes: a consensus approach. *Am J Kidney Dis* 36:646–661, 2000

Bhattacharyya A, Brown S, Hughes S, Vice PA: Insulin lispro and regular insulin in pregnancy. *QJM* 94:255–260, 2001

Biesenbach G, Grafinger P, Stoger H, Zarzgornik J: How pregnancy influences renal function in nephropathic type 1 diabetic women depends on their preconceptional creatinine clearance. *J Nephrol* 12:41–46, 1999

Bolli GB, Perriello G, Fanelli C, De Feo P: Nocturnal blood glucose control in type 1 diabetes mellitus. *Diabetes Care* 16 (Suppl. 3):71–89, 1993

Brunelle BL, Llewelyn J, Anderson JH Jr, Gale EA, Koivisto VA: Meta-analysis of the effect of insulin lispro on severe hypoglycemia in patients with type 1 diabetes. *Diabetes Care* 21:1726–1731, 1998

Chew EY, Mills JL, Metzger BE, Remaley NA, Jovanovic L, Knopp RH, Conley M, Rand L, Simpson JL, Holmes LB, et al.: Metabolic control and progression of retinopathy: The Diabetes in Early Pregnancy Study: National Institute of Child Health and Human Development Diabetes in Early Pregnancy Study. *Diabetes Care* 18:631–637, 1995

Ciaraldi TP, Carter L, Seipke G, Mudaliar S, Henry RR: Effects of the long-acting insulin glargine on cultured human skeletal muscle cells: comparisons to insulin and IGF-1. *J Clin Endocrinol Metab* 86:5838–5847, 2001

Colombel A, Murat A, Krempf M, Kuchly-Anton B, Charbonnel B: Improvement of blood glucose control in type 1 diabetic patients treated with lispro and multiple NPH injections. *Diabet Med* 16:319–324, 1999

Combs CA, Rosenn B, Kitzmiller JL, Khoury JC, Wheeler BC, Miuodovnik M: Early-pregnancy proteinuria in diabetes related to preeclampsia. *Obstet Gynecol* 82:802–807, 1993

Coustan DR, Berkowitz RL, Hobbins JC: Tight metabolic control of overt diabetes in pregnancy. *Am J Med* 68:845–852, 1980

Del Sindaco P, Ciofetta M, Lalli C, Perriello G, Pampanelli S, Torlone E, Brunetti P, Bolli GB: Use of the short-acting insulin analogue lispro in intensive treatment of type 1 diabetes mellitus: importance of appropriate replacement of basal insulin and time-interval injection-meal. *Diabet Med* 15:592–600, 1998

Diabetes Control and Complications Trial Research Group: Effect of pregnancy on microvascular complications in the Diabetes Control and Complications Trial. *Diabetes Care* 23:1084–1091, 2000

Dietary Guidelines for Americans, 2010. United States Department of Agriculture, Center for Nutrition Policy and Promotion. http://www.cnpp.usda.gov/DGAs2010-PolicyDocument.htm. Accessed 5 September 2012

Ebeling P, Jansson PA, Smith U, Lalli C, Bolli GB, Koivisto VA: Strategies toward improved control during insulin lispro therapy in IDDM: importance of basal insulin. *Diabetes Care* 20:1287–1289, 1997

Eidem I, Stene LC, Henriksen T, Hanssen KF, Vangen S, Vollset SE, Joner G: Congenital anomalies in newborns of women with type 1 diabetes: nationwide population-based study in Norway, 1999–2004. *Acta Obstet Gynecol Scand* 89:1403–1411, 2010

Elman KD, Welch RA, Frank RN, Goyert G, Sokol RJ: Diabetic retinopathy in pregnancy: a review. *Obstet Gynecol* 75:119–127, 1990

Evers IM, de Valk HW, Visser GH: Risk of complications of pregnancy in women with type 1 diabetes: nationwide prospective study in the Netherlands. *BMJ* doi:10.1136/bmj.38043.583160.EE (published 5 April 2004)

Freinkel N, Lewis NJ, Akazawa S, Roth S, Forman L: The honeybee syndrome: implications of the teratogenicity of mannose in rat-embryo culture. *N Engl J Med* 310:223–230, 1984

Führmann K, Reiher H, Semmler K, Glockner E: The effect of intensified conventional insulin therapy before and during pregnancy on the malformation rate in offspring of diabetic mothers. *Exp Clin Endocrinol* 83:173–177, 1984

Garg SK, Frias JP, Anil S, Gottlieb PA, Mackenzie T, Jackson WE: Insulin lispro therapy in pregnancies complicated by diabetes type 1: glycemic control and maternal and fetal outcomes. *Endocr Pract* 9:187–193, 2003

Greene MF: Prevention and diagnosis of congenital anomalies in diabetic pregnancy. *Clin Perinatol* 20:533–547, 1993

Greene MF, Hare JW, Cloherty JP, Benacerraf BR, Soeldner JS: First-trimester hemoglobin A1 and risk for major malformation and spontaneous abortion in diabetic pregnancy. *Teratology* 39:225–231, 1989

Guerin A, Nisenbaum R, Ray JG: Use of maternal GHb concentration to estimate the risk of congenital anomalies in the offspring of women with prepregnancy diabetes. *Diabetes Care* 30:1920–1925, 2007 [online appendix 2]

Hansson L, Zanchetti A, Carruthers SG, Dahlof B, Elmfeldt D, Julius S, Menard J, Rahn KH, Wedel H, Westerling S: Effects of intensive blood pressure lowering and low-dose aspirin in patients with hypertension: principal results of the Hypertension Optimal Treatment (HOT randomized trial: The HOT Study Group). *Lancet* 351:1755–1762, 1998

Hare JW, White P: Pregnancy in diabetes complicated by vascular disease. *Diabetes* 26:953–955, 1977

Henricsson M, Berntorp K, Berntorp E, Fernlund P, Sundkvist G: Progression of retinopathy after improved metabolic control in type 2 diabetic patients: relation to IGF-1 and hemostatic variables. *Diabetes Care* 22:1944–1949, 1999

Idama TO, Lindow SW, French M, Masson EA: Preliminary experience with the use of insulin lispro in pregnant diabetic women. *J Obstet Gynecol* 21:350–351, 2001

Institute of Medicine Food and Nutrition Board: *Dietary Reference Intakes: The Essential Guide to Nutrient Requirements.* Washington, DC, National Academies Press, 2006

Johnstone FO, Hepburn DA, Smith AF: Can prepregnancy care of diabetic women reduce the risk of abnormal babies? *BMJ* 301:1070–1074, 1990

Jovanovic L, Druzin M, Peterson CM: Effect of euglycemia on the outcome of pregnancy in insulin dependent diabetic women as compared with normal control subjects. *Am J Med* 71:921–927, 1982

Jovanovic L, Druzin M, Peterson CM: The effect of euglycemia on the outcome of pregnancy in insulin-dependent diabetics as compared to normal controls. *Am J Med* 71:921–927, 1981

Jovanovic L, Ilic S, Pettitt DJ, Hugo K, Gutierrez M, Bowsher RR, Bastyr EJ 3rd: Metabolic and immunologic effects of insulin lispro in gestational diabetes. *Diabetes Care* 22:1422–1427, 1999

Jovanovic L, Peterson CM: De novo hypothyroidism in pregnancies complicated by type I diabetes and proteinuria: a new syndrome. *Am J Obstet Gynecol* 159:441–446, 1988

Jovanovic L, Peterson CM, Saxena BB, Dawood MY, Saudek CD: Feasibility of maintaining euglycemia in insulin-dependent diabetic women. *Am J Med* 68:105–112, 1980

Kalter H, Warkany J: Congenital malformations: etiologic factors and their role in prevention. *N Engl J Med* 308:424–431, 1983

Khoury JC, Miodovnik M, LeMasters G, Sibai B: Pregnancy outcome and progression of diabetic nephropathy. What's next? *J Maternal Fetal Neonatal Med* 11: 238–244, 2002

Kimmerle R, Heinemann L, Delecki A, Berger M: Severe hypoglycemia: incidence and predisposing factors in 85 pregnancies of type 1 diabetic women. *Diabetes Care* 15:1034–1037, 1992

Kitzmiller JL, Cloherty JP, Younger MD, Tabatabaii A, Rothchild S, Sosenko I, Epstein M, Sinah S, Neff R: Diabetic pregnancy and perinatal outcome. *Am J Obstet Gynecol* 131:560–580, 1978

Kitzmiller JL, Gavin LA, Gin GD, Jovanovic-Peterson L, Main EK, Zigrang WD: Preconception care of diabetes: glycemic control prevents congenital anomalies. *JAMA* 265:731–736, 1991

Kurtzhals P, Schaffer L, Sorensen A, Kristensen C, Jonassen I, Schmid C, Trüb T: Correlations of receptor binding and metabolic and mitogenic potencies of insulin analogs designed for clinical use. *Diabetes* 49:999–1005, 2000

Lazarus JM, Bourgoignie JJ, Buckalew VM, Green T, Levey AS, Milas NC, Paranandi L, Peterson JC, Porash JG, Rauch S, Soucie HM, Stollar C: Achievement and safety of a low BP goal in chronic renal disease: The Modification of Diet in Renal Disease Study Group. *Hypertension* 29:641–650, 1997

Lepore M, Pampanelli S, Fanelli C, Porcellati F, Bartocci L, Di Vincenzo A, Cordoni C, Costa E, Brunetti P, Bolli GM: Pharmacokinetics and pharmacodynamics of subcutaneous injection of long-acting human insulin analog glargine, NPH insulin and ultralente human insulin and continuous subcutaneous infusion of insulin lispro. *Diabetes* 49:2142–2148, 2000

Loukovaara S, Immonen I, Teramo KA, Kaaja R: Progression of retinopathy during pregnancy in type 1 diabetic women treated with insulin lispro. *Diabetes Care* 26:1193–1198, 2003

Macintosh MC, Fleming KM, Bailey JA, Doyle P, Modder J, Acolet D, Golightly S, Miller A: Perinatal mortality and congenital anomalies in babies of women with type 1 or type 2 diabetes in England, Wales, and Northern Ireland: population based study. *BMJ* doi:10.1136/bmj.38856.692986.AE (published 16 June 2006)

Masson EA, Patmore JE, Brash PD, Baxter M, Caldwell G, Gallen AW, Price PA, Vice PA, Walker JD, Lindow SW: Pregnancy outcome in type 1 diabetes mellitus treated with insulin lispro (Humalog). *Diabet Med* 20:46–50, 2003

Mathiesen ER, Hod M, Ivanisevic M, et al., on behalf of the Detemir in Pregnancy Study Group: Maternal efficacy and safety outcomes in a randomized, controlled trial comparing insulin detemir with NPH insulin in 310 pregnant women with type 1 diabetes. *Diabetes Care* 2012; epublished 30 July 2012 doi:10.2337/dc11-2264

McCance DR, Damm P, Mathiesen ER, Hod M, Kaaja R, Dunne F, Jensen LE, Mersebach H: Evaluation of insulin antibodies and placental transfer of insulin aspart in pregnant women with type 1 diabetes mellitus. *Diabetologia* 51:2141–2143, 2008

Mecacci F, Carignani L, Cioni R, Bartoli E, Parretti E, La Torre P, Scarselli G, Mello G: Maternal metabolic control and perinatal outcome in women with gestational diabetes treated with regular or lispro insulin: comparison with non-diabetic pregnant women. *Eur J Obste Gynecol Reprod Biol* 111:19–24, 2003

Miller E, Hare JW, Cloherty JP, Dunn PH, Gleason RE, Soeldner JS, Kitzmiller JL: Elevated maternal hemoglobin A1c in early pregnancy and major congenital anomalies in infants of diabetic mothers. *N Engl J Med* 304:1331–1134, 1981

Mills JL, Baker L, Goldman AS: Malformations in infants of diabetic mothers occur before the seventh gestational week: implications for treatment. *Diabetes* 28:292–293, 1979

Miodovnik M, Lavin JP, Knowles HC, Holroyde J, Stys S: Spontaneous abortion among insulin-dependent diabetic women. *Am J Obstet Gynecol* 150:372–375, 1984

Ochsenbein-Kolble N, Roos M, Gasser T, Huch R, Zimmermann R: Cross sectional study of automated blood pressure measurements throughout pregnancy. *Br J Obstet Gynaecol* 111:319–325, 2004

Persson B, Swahn M, Hjertberg R, Hanson U, Nord E, Nordlander E, Hansson LO: Insulin lispro therapy in pregnancies complicated by type 1 diabetes mellitus. *Diabetes Res Clin Pract* 58:115–121, 2002

Peterson CM, Jovanovic-Peterson L, Mills JL, Conley MR, Knopp RH, Reed GF, Aarons JH, Holmes LB, Brown Z, Van Allen M, Schmeltz R, Metzger BE, the National Institute of Child Health and Human Development–The Diabetes in Early Pregnancy Study: Changes in cholesterol, triglycerides, body weight, and blood pressure. *Am J Obstet Gynecol* 166:513–518, 1992

Pettitt DJ, Ospina P, Kolaczynski JW, Jovanovic L: Comparison of an insulin analog, insulin aspart, and regular human insulin with no insulin in gestational diabetes mellitus. *Diabetes Care* 26:183–186, 2003

Phelps RL, Sakol P, Metzger BE, Jampol LM, Freinkel N: Changes in diabetic retinopathy during pregnancy: correlations with regulation of hyper-glycemia. *Arch Ophthalmol* 104:1806–1810, 1986

Philipson EH, Super DM: Gestational diabetes mellitus: does it recur in subsequent pregnancy? *Am J Obstet Gynecol* 160:1324–1331, 1989

Pollex EK, Feig DS, Lubetsky A, Yip PM, Koren G: Insulin glargine safety in pregnancy: a transplacental transfer study. *Diabetes Care* 33:29–33, 2010

Purdy LP, Hantsch CE, Molitch ME, Metzger BE, Phelps RL, Dooley SL, et al.: Effect of pregnancy on renal function in patients with moderate-to-severe diabetic renal insufficiency. *Diabetes Care* 19:1067–1074, 1996

Reece EA, Gabriella S, Abdalla M: The prevention of diabetes associated birth defects. *Semin Perinatol* 12:292–302, 1988

Reece EA, Hobbins JS: Diabetic embryopathy: pathogenesis, prenatal diagnosis and prevention. *Obstet Gynecol Surv* 41:325–335, 1986

Sadler TW, Hunter ES, Wynn RE, Phillips LH: Evidence for multifactorial origin of diabetes-induced embryopathies. *Diabetes* 38:70–74, 1989

Sheth BP: Does pregnancy accelerate the rate of progression of diabetic retinopathy? *Curr Diab Rep* 2:327–330, 2002

Steel JM: Personal experience of prepregnancy care in women with insulin dependent diabetes. *Aust NZ J Obstet Gynaecol* 34:135–139, 1994

Steel JM: Prepregnancy counseling and contraception in the insulin-dependent diabetic patient. *Clin Obstet Gynecol* 28:553–568, 1985

UK Prospective Diabetes Study Group: Tight blood pressure control and risk of macrovascular and microvascular complications in type 2 diabetes: UKPDS 38. *BMJ* 317:703–713, 1998

Von Dadelszen P, Ornstein MP, Bull SB, Logan AG, Koren G, Magee LA: Fall in mean arterial pressure and fetal growth restriction in pregnancy hypertension: a meta-analysis. *Lancet* 355:87–92, 2000

Wahabi HA, Alzeidan RA, Bawazeer GA, Alansari LA, Esmaeil SA: Preconception care for diabetic women for improving maternal and fetal outcomes: a systematic review and meta-analysis. *BMC Pregnancy Childbirth* 10:63, 2010

Warram JH, Martin BC, Krowlewski AS: Risk of IDDM in children of diabetic mothers decreases with increasing maternal age at pregnancy. *Diabetes* 40:1679–1684, 1991

Wyatt JW, Frias JL, Hoyme HE, Jovanovic L, Kaaja R, Brown F, Garg S, Lee-Parritz A, Seely EW, Kerr L, Mattoo V, Tan M, IONS Study Group: Congenital anomaly rate in offspring of mothers with type 1 diabetes treated with insulin lispro during pregnancy. *Diabet Med* 21:2001–2007, 2004

Ylinen K, Aula P, Stenman U-H, Kesaniemi-Kuokkanea T, Teramo K: Risk of minor and major fetal malformations in diabetics with high haemoglobin A1c values in early pregnancy. *BMJ* 289:345–346, 1984

# Contraception in Women with Diabetes and Prediabetes: Options and Assessing Risk and Benefits

# Highlights
## Contraception in Women with Diabetes and Prediabetes: Options and Assessing Risk and Benefits

■ Use of a safe and efficacious contraceptive method is integral to avoid unplanned pregnancy in women with diabetes who are in poor glycemic control and is necessary to plan a pregnancy in women who are in good glycemic control and optimal health. When counseling women, comorbid conditions associated with diabetes must be considered as well as the woman's lifestyle, individual preferences, and ease of use.

■ Standard guidelines recommended to monitor glycemic control, serum lipid levels, blood pressure, and renal and retinal surveillance should be evaluated and considered when prescribing contraceptives in all women with diabetes or prediabetes.

■ Women with prior gestational diabetes mellitus (GDM) and normal postpartum glucose tolerance can use all methods of contraception (Category 1). Progestin-only methods in women with prior GDM who are breast-feeding should be avoided.

■ The copper-medicated intrauterine devices are metabolically neutral and have been shown to be highly efficacious in women with diabetes and other comorbidities and have no restrictions in their use (Category 1). They do not increase risks of pelvic inflammatory disease.

■ Estrogen-containing methods, including combination oral contraceptives, vaginal rings, and transdermal patches, should not be prescribed in women with diabetic sequelae (retinopathy, nephropathy, or neuropathy), hypertension or other cardiovascular disease, or increased coagulation risk, or in any women during the first 6 weeks after delivery.

■ Progestin-only methods, including progestin-only oral contraceptives, injectables, subcutaneous implants, and progestin-releasing intrauterine devices (IUD), do not affect blood pressure levels or coagulation factors and have minimal lipid metabolic effects. These methods can be considered as acceptable methods (Category 2).

■ Once childbearing is completed, permanent sterilization of the woman with diabetes is a highly efficacious method to prevent unplanned pregnancy and can be accomplished via surgical ligation or hysteroscopic surgical tubal occlusion.

# Contraception in Women with Diabetes and Prediabetes: Options and Assessing Risk and Benefits

When counseling and providing contraceptives, the health-care provider must consider not only the general risks and benefits of contraceptive methods but also their metabolic effects on diabetes and existing comorbidites when counseling and prescribing contraceptives. Equally important is the consequence of an unplanned pregnancy for the woman and her potential offspring. Should pregnancy occur in the presence of poor metabolic control, the likelihood of major congenital anomalies is ~20–23% (Miller 1981). Effective contraception allows a woman and her physician to plan pregnancy when glycemic control is achieved (A1C <7%), reducing the risk of anomalies and permitting her health status to be optimized with respect to hypertension and microvascular disease, and reducing her risks for pregnancy complications. Women with a history of gestational diabetes mellitus (GDM) should be tested 6 weeks postpartum and at least every 3 years for diabetes as ~50–60% will develop diabetes within 5–20 years of their index pregnancy (Trussell 2007). Women with prior GDM are at risk for or share many of the same comorbidities found in women with diabetes (e.g., metabolic syndrome, obesity, hypertension, and hyperlipidemia). These comorbidities and the presence of diabetic sequelae must be considered when planning a pregnancy or selecting a contraceptive method. Standard guidelines recommended to monitor glycemic control, serum lipid levels, blood pressure, and renal and retinal surveillance should be evaluated and considered when prescribing contraceptives in all women with diabetes or prediabetes.

Equally important as the method selection is the patient's acceptance of side effects, her comfort with the method, and her ability to successfully use her chosen method. The practitioner's goal is to prescribe the method that poses the least risk relating to her diabetic disease process, has the greatest efficacy, and is acceptable to the woman. Second, although the method may not be risk free, individualized counseling, lifestyle interventions, and adequate control of her disease process generally can minimize these risks to an acceptable level. This chapter will deal with methods with higher efficacy (Trussell 2007), primarily hormonal methods and intrauterine devices. Barrier methods, including spermicides, diaphragm, condoms, cervical caps, and contraceptive sponge, will not be considered in detail as there are no medical contraindications to their use except higher failure (Table 2.1).

## INTRAUTERINE DEVICES

The guidelines for use of intrauterine devices (IUDs) in women with diabetes follow the same guidelines as in healthy women—for example, those who are parous and at low risk for and without a recent history of sexually transmitted diseases or pelvic inflammatory disease (PID). The copper-medicated IUD (Cu-IUD) is an excellent choice. It is metabolically neutral and offers pregnancy protection for 10 years. In a large meta-analysis of several prospective World Health Organization (WHO) trials, the overall incidence of PID associated with Cu-IUD, use was 1.6 per 1,000 women-years of IUD use (U.S. Medical Eligibility Criteria for Contraceptive Use, 2010). One drawback is an increased menstrual blood loss, which can be counteracted by daily iron supplementation or multivitamins and minerals. In several high-risk populations, including women with type 1 diabetes (T1D) or type 2 diabetes (T2D), no IUD-associated increase in PID has been found and thus is given a U.S. Medical Eligibility Criteria for Contraceptive Use (U.S.M.E.C. 2010) Risk Category of 1 (Table 2.2) (Wiese 1977, Gosen 1982, Skouby 1984, Farley 1992, Kimmerle 1993, Kjos 1994).

Mirena®, the levonorgestrel-containing intrauterine system (LNG-IUS), is both an IUD and a progestin method with a 5-year efficacy. The LNG-IUS releases ~10% of the dose and reaches 5% of the plasma level of a 105-mcg dose of oral LNG. Thus, its systemic metabolic effect appears to be minimal, but it does exert a local progestin effect on the endometrium, decreasing menstrual blood loss. Its advantages include lower pregnancy rates and lower rates of PID but it entails greater rates of discontinuation because of hormonal side effects. It is an excellent choice for women with diabetes who have heavy menses or who are at risk for endometrial hyperplasia (e.g., obese, oligomenorrhea, or polycystic ovarian syndrome). Two recent 1-year, randomized control trials comparing the use of Cu-IUD with LGN-IUD in women with T1D and T2D showed no effect on glycemic control, insulin dosage, hemocoagulation, fibrinolysis, or cholesterol levels. The 2011 U.S.M.E.C. retained the LNG-IUS in women with diabetes and associated comorbidities as Category 2, with the advantages generally outweighing theoretical or proven risks based on the small number of studies to date.

## HORMONAL CONTRACEPTIVES

Hormonal contraceptives can be delivered via several routes, in several formulations and varying dosage. Decisions about whether or not to prescribe hormonal contraceptives and which method is appropriate to prescribe can be made using a series of questions.

### QUESTION 1: IS THE WOMAN A CANDIDATE FOR HORMONAL CONTRACEPTION?

Reproductive-age women produce estrogen and progesterone, and it is not surprising that most women can safely use hormonal contraception. Exceptions in which hormonal contraception are contraindicated include women with *1*) liver disease that interferes with liver metabolism of steroids, for example, active hepatitis or cirrhosis (nonalcoholic fatty liver disease); *2)* cholestasis associated with prior hormonal contraception use; *3)* malignant or benign liver tumors; and *4)* estrogen- or progesterone-sensitive malignancies.

## QUESTION 2: IS THE WOMAN A CANDIDATE FOR ESTROGEN-CONTAINING CONTRACEPTION?

Estrogen itself does not provide contraception, but it helps in cycle control when given in combination with progestins. Estrogen-plus-progestin methods are most widely prescribed as combination oral contraceptives (COC), but they also are available transdermally (Evra® Patch and vaginal NuvaRing®) or via monthly combination injectable contraceptives (CIC), which currently are off the market. The estrogen component also produces a dose-dependent increase in liver-produced globulins, thereby increasing coagulation factors, the risk for a thrombotic event, angiotensin II levels, and mean arterial blood pressure (Meade 1982, Godsland 1990). There is generally a desirable effect on serum lipid levels (lowering low-density lipoprotein cholesterol, increasing high-density lipoprotein cholesterol) and mild increase in triglycerides. These effects are mediated largely through the first pass through the liver, after absorption from the gut. Notably, estrogen has no effect on insulin resistance. Therefore, women with diabetes who have vascular sequelae, hypertension, or cardiovascular disease (or if they smoke or have prior thrombotic disease) should not use estrogen-containing contraceptives and the U.S.M.E.C. has assigned a Category 3/4 risk for these conditions irrespective of the delivery route.

Women with prior GDM or diabetes without vascular disease or hypertension are candidates for combination methods either as COC via the Evra® Patch or vaginal NuvaRing®. The U.S.M.E.C. has assigned COC use a Category 2 risk in women with diabetes who do not have vascular disease and a Category 1 risk in women with prior GDM based on studies showing no increase in risk of developing diabetes with COC use. Studies have also shown no increased risk in the development of diabetes with low-dose COC use in women with prior GDM (Skouby 1985, 1987; Kjos 1990, 1998).

When selecting a COC, the formulations with the lowest possible dose or potency of both estrogen (20–35 mcg) and progestin should be selected as a general rule. This strategy has been supported in several short-term or prospective studies in women with T1D who were followed for up to 1 year with lower doses of the older progestins, including norethindrone (≤0.75 mg mean daily dose), or triphasic levonorgestrel preparation; and the newer progestins, including gestodene or desogestrel. All formulations were found to have minimal effect on diabetic control, lipid metabolism, and cardiovascular risk factors. Retrospective, cross-sectional studies and case-control trials in women with T1D have not found any increased risk of or progression of diabetic sequelae (retinopathy, renal disease, or hypertension) with past or current use of oral contraceptives.

Currently, it is unclear whether transdermal patches, vaginal rings, or monthly injections offer a metabolic advantage over COC. Small studies examining the vaginal ring in healthy women and in women with T1D have found no difference compared to control subjects or in women with T1D using COC, in glucose metabolism, lipids levels, or hemostasis (Kimmerle 1993, Grigoryan, 2008). Thus the route of combination contraceptives should be based on patient preference, expected reliability in administration of method (daily, weekly, or monthly), and reversibility (greater delay in return of fertility with CIC, currently off the market).

## QUESTION 3: WHAT IS THE BEST DOSE AND FORMULATION OF ORAL PROGESTIN IF THE WOMAN IS A CANDIDATE FOR COC?

COC contain a wide variety of progestin formulations and doses. Most progestins are testosterone derivatives and have varying degrees of androgenic effects (e.g., decreasing sex-binding globulin, increasing insulin resistance, and causing adverse changes in serum lipids). Newer formulations of oral progestins (desogestrel, gestodene, drospirenone) with decreased androgenicity or older lower-dose and -potency norethindrone minimize androgenic side effects and therefore generally should be selected (Speroff 1993). Consideration of which COC formulation to prescribe is especially important in women in whom increased insulin resistance, unfavorable lipid profiles, and hirsutism should be minimized (e.g., diabetes, prior gestational diabetes, metabolic syndrome, and polycystic ovarian syndrome).

If women are not able to use estrogen, and yet desire a hormonal method, most will be candidates for progestin-only methods. Importantly, for women with hypertension, cardiovascular disease, and risk of thrombosis, progestin-only formulations do not affect liver globulin production and thereby do not increase blood pressure or coagulation factors (Meade 1982, Wilson 1984).

## QUESTION 4: WHAT IS THE IDEAL ROUTE OF ADMINISTRATION OF PROGESTIN-ONLY CONTRACEPTION?

Progestin-only methods can be delivered orally (PO-OC) or via injection, as implants, or via the uterine cavity (IUD). There are two formulations of PO-OC, one containing norethindrone (0.35 mg daily) and the other containing levonorgestrel (0.75 mg daily); both are taken daily with no placebo periods.

Alternative longer-acting routes of progestin-only contraception include injections, given every 3 months (depo-medroxyprogesterone acetate, DMPA) or subcutaneous implants (etonogestrel) every 3 years. The levonorgestrel implant (Norplant®) is no longer marketed and has been replaced by the etonorgestrel implants Implanon® and then Nexplanon®. Currently, minimal literature exists comparing metabolic effects in healthy or high-risk women to distinguish among the various doses and routes of progestins. One small study showed no significant metabolic changes on glucose, lipids, albuminuria, or retinal vasculature over 2 years in insulin-treated women using the etonorgestrel implant (Vicente 2008). DMPA has in several studies been shown to have more adverse effects on lipids and insulin resistance compared with Norplant® in healthy women (Fajumi 1983, Deslypere 1985, Liew 1985, Fahraeus 1986, Haiba 1989, Fahmy 1991, Xiang 2006). DMPA also has a longer return of fertility after discontinuation and has been associated with weight gain in normal women and women with diabetes. Thus DMPA is not a first-line progestin agent for women with cardiovascular disease and risk factors, including coronary artery disease, history of stroke, diabetes with vascular disease, polycystic ovarian syndrome, and obesity (Category 3).

## Table 2.1 Percentage of Women Experiencing an Unintended Pregnancy during the First Year of Typical Use and Perfect Use and the Percentage Continuing Use at the End of the First year in the U.S.

| Method | Typical Use | Perfect Use | Continuation at 1 Year |
|---|---|---|---|
| **Low Efficacy** | | | |
| No method | 85% | 85% | 43% |
| Withdrawal | 27% | 4% | -- |
| Fertility awareness | 25% | 3–5% | 51% |
| **Barrier Methods** | | | |
| Spermicides | 29% | 18% | 42% |
| Vaginal sponge (parous/nullip) | 32%/16% | 20%/9% | 46%/56% |
| Diaphragm | 16% | 6% | 57% |
| Male condom | 15% | 2% | 53% |
| **Estrogen/Progestin Methods** | | | |
| Combination oral contraceptives (COC) | 8% | 0.3% | 68% |
| Transdermal patch (Evra®) | 8% | 0.3% | 68% |
| Vaginal ring (NuvaRing®) | 8% | 0.3% | 68% |
| **Progestin-Only Methods** | | | |
| Progestin-only oral contraceptive (PO-OC) | 8% | 0.3% | 68% |
| LNG-IUS (Mirena®) | 0.2% | 0.2% | 80% |
| DMPA injection (Depo-Provera®) | 3% | 0.3% | 56% |
| Implant (Implanon®) | 0.05% | 0.05% | 84% |
| **Nonhormonal** | | | |
| Copper-medicated IUD (Paragard®) | 0.8% | 0.6% | 78% |
| **Sterilization** | | | |
| Bilateral tubal ligation Essure® | 0.5% | 0.5% | 100% |

Adapted from Trussell J: Contraceptive efficacy. In *Contraceptive Technology*. 19th ed. Hatcher RA, Ed. New York, NY, Ardent Media, 2008, p. 19–41.

Oral progestins have the advantage of being more widely studied and have a better-documented safety profile. Women are able to rapidly discontinue therapy if side effects occur, and this can be useful when given as trial therapy to see whether women can tolerate progestin side effects before administering a longer-acting injectable or implant progestin. Without clearly demonstrated metabolic differences, the various routes of administration can be tailored to a woman's lifestyle, convenience, and reliability.

Several short-term studies of T1D women have shown little to no metabolic effect of the norethindrone PO-OC on glucose and lipid metabolism. In postpartum Latina women with previous GDM who were breast-feeding, the use of PO-OC was associated with a threefold adjusted increased risk of developing T2D compared with non–breast-feeding women with previous GDM using COC

(Kjos 1998). This effect was duration dependent, with women using PO-OC >8 months having nearly a sixfold increased risk. Thus, it is prudent for these women to either use barrier methods while lactating or wait until 6 weeks after delivery to begin a COC. Similar caution is advised in prescribing DMPA to postpartum breast-feeding women with previous GDM compared with non–breast-feeding women with prior GDM, for whom the risk of developing diabetes was increased twofold (Xiang 2006). Minimal or no metabolic effect on blood pressure or lipids was seen on long-term use of DMPA in women with prior GDM.

## PERMANENT STERILIZATION

For the individual with diabetes who has completed childbearing, permanent surgical sterilization of either the woman or her mate offers a reasonable contraceptive option. Sterilization can be done surgically via laproscopy or minilaparotomy. An excellent alternative is Essure®, in which flexible coils are inserted into the fallopian tubes via hysteroscopy, which causes tubal scarring and occlusion after 3 months. A hysterosalpingogram is performed at 3 months to document tubal occlusion. This method avoids general anesthesia and surgery and is done as an office procedure. The pregnancy rate after surgical sterilization of the woman (or man) is <0.5%. Those pregnancies that do occur in sterilized women, however, are more likely to be ectopically implanted. Consideration in counseling should be given to the fact that women with diabetes are at increased risk with future pregnancies, whereas their spouses or significant others are not. If male surgical sterilization has been carried out, and the marriage or relationship should dissolve in the future, the women with diabetes would still be susceptible to pregnancy.

**Table 2.2 Contraception Options for Women with Diabetes and Other Associated Conditions and Assessment of Risks Based on the U.S. Medical Eligibility Criteria for Contraceptive Use**

| Condition | Subcondition | Estrogen Plus Progestin | Progestin-Only Oral Contraception | Injection | Implant | LNG-IUD | Copper-IUD |
|---|---|---|---|---|---|---|---|
| Diabetes | Hx of Gestational Diabetes | 1 | 1 | 1 | 1 | 1 | 1 |
| No vascular disease | | | | | | | |
| | Type 1 | 2 | 2 | 2 | 2 | 2 | 1 |
| | Type 2 | 2 | 2 | 2 | 2 | 2 | 1 |

| Condition | Subcondition | Estrogen Plus Progestin | Progestin-Only Oral Contraception | Injection | Implant | LNG-IUD | Copper-IUD |
|---|---|---|---|---|---|---|---|
| Vascular disease or diabetes for >20 years duration | | | | | | | |
| | Nephropathy, retinopathy, neuropathy | 3 / 4* | 2 | 3 | 2 | 2 | 1 |
| | Other vascular disease or >20 years duration | 3 / 4* | 2 | 3 | 2 | 2 | 1 |
| Hyperlipidemia | | 2 /3 * | 2* | 2* | 2* | 2* | 1 |
| Hypertension | | | | | | | |
| History high blood pressure in pregnancy | | 2 | 1 | 1 | 1 | 1 | 1 |
| Adequately controlled | | 3* | 1* | 2* | 1* | 1 | 1 |
| Elevated blood pressure levels | | | | | | | |
| | Systolic 140–159 mmHg or diastolic 90–99 mmHg | 3 | 1 | 2 | 1 | 1 | 1 |
| | Systolic ≥160 mmHg or diastolic ≥100 mmHg | 4 | 2 | 3 | 2 | 2 | 1 |
| Obesity | BMI ≥30 kg/m² | 2 | 1 | 1 | 1 | 1 | 1 |
| | Menarch to 18 years and BMI ≥30 kg/m² | 2 | 1 | 2 | 1 | 1 | 1 |
| History of Bariatric Surgery | | | | | | | |
| Restrictive procedures | | 1 | 1 | 1 | 1 | 1 | 1 |
| Malabsorptive procedures | | COC: 3 Patch/Ring:1 | 3 | 1 | 1 | 1 | 1 |
| Endometrial Hyperplasia | | 1 | 1 | 1 | 1 | 1 | 1 |
| Postpartum | | | | | | | |
| <21 days | | 4 | 1 | 1 | 1 | | |
| 21–42 days | | | | | | | |
| | With other risk factors for VTE | 3 | 1 | 1 | 1 | | |
| | Without other risk factors for VTE | 2 | 1 | 1 | 1 | | |
| >42 days | | 1 | 1 | 1 | 1 | 1 | 1 |
| Postpartum breast-feeding or non–breast-feeding or post–cesarean section | 10 min to <4 weeks after delivery | | | | | 2 | 2 |
| | ≥4 weeks postpartum | | | | | 1 | 1 |
| | Puerpal sepsis | | | | | 4 | 4 |

Key to risk categories: 1, No restriction (method can be used); 2, Advantages generally outweigh theoretical or proven risks; 3, Theoretical or proven risks usually outweigh the advantages; 4, Unacceptable health risk (method not to be used).

*Please see the complete guidance for a clarification to this classification: www.cdc.gov/reproductivehealth/unintendedpregnancy/USMEC.htm.

From "U.S. Medical Eligibility Criteria for Contraceptive Use, 2010." *MMWR* 59:1–tt85, 2010.

## SELECTED READINGS

Committee Opinion no. 505: Understanding and using the U.S. Medical Eligibility Criteria for Contraceptive Use, 2010. *Obstet Gynecol* 118:754–760, 2011

Damm P, Mathiesen ER, Petersen KR, Kjos S: Contraception after GDM. *Diabetes Care* 30 (Suppl. 2):S200–S205, 2007

Grigoryan OG, Grodnitskaya EE, Andreeva EN, Shestakova MV, Melnichenko GA, Dedov II: Contraception in perimenopausal women with diabetes mellitus. *Contraception* 22:198–206, 2006

## REFERENCES

Deslypere JP, Thiery N, Vermeulen A: Effect of long-term hormonal contraception in plasma lipids. *Contraception* 31:633–642, 1985

Fahmy K, Abdel-Razik, Shaaraway M, et al.: Effect of long-acting progestagen-only injectable contraceptives on carbohydrate metabolism and its hormonal profile. *Contraception* 44:419–429, 1991

Fahraeus L, Sydsjo A, Wallentin L: Lipoprotein changes during treatment of pelvic endometriosis with medroxyprogesterone acetate. *Fert Steril* 45:501–506, 1986

Farley TMM, Rosenberg MJ, Rowe PJ, Chen J-H, Meirek O: Intrauterine devices and pelvic inflammatory disease: an international perspective. *Lancet* 339:785–788, 1992

Fajumi JO: Alterations in blood lipids and side effects induced by depo-provera in Nigerian women. *Contraception* 27:161–175, 1983

Godsland IF, Crook D, Simpson R, et al.: The effects of different formulations of oral contraceptive agents on lipid and carbohydrate metabolism. *N Engl J Med* 323:1375–1381, 1990

Gosen C, Steel J, Ross A, Springerbett A: Intrauterine contraception in diabetic women. *Lancet* 1:530–535, 1982

Grigoryan OG, Grodnitskaya EE, Andreeva EN, Chebotnikova TV, Melnichenko GA: Use of the NuvaRing hormone-releasing system in late reproductive-age women with type 2 diabetes mellitus. *Gynecological Endocrinology* 24:99–104, 2008

Haiba NA, et al.: Clinical evaluation of two monthly injectable contraceptives and their effects on some metabolic parameters. *Contraception* 39:619–632, 1989

Kimmerle R, Weiss R, Berger M, Kurz K-H: Effectiveness, safety and acceptability of a copper intrauterine device (CU Safe 300) in type I diabetic women. *Diabetes Care* 16:1227–1230, 1993

Kjos SL, Ballagh SA, La Cour M, Xiang A, Mishell DR Jr: The copper T380A intrauterine device in women with type II diabetes mellitus. *Obstet Gynecol* 84:1006–1009, 1994

Kjos SL, Peters RK, Xiang A, Thomas D, Schaefer U, Buchanan TA: Contraception and the risk of type 2 diabetes mellitus in Latina women with prior gestational diabetes mellitus. *JAMA* 280:533–538, 1998

Kjos SL, Shoupe D, Douyan S, et al.: Effect of low-dose oral contraceptives on carbohydrate and lipid metabolism in women with recent gestational diabetes: results of a controlled, randomized, prospective study. *Am J Obstet Gynecol* 163:1822–1827, 1990

Liew DFM, Ng CSA, Yong YM, et al.: Long term effects of depo-provera on carbohydrate and lipid metabolism. *Contraception* 31:51–64, 1985

Meade TW: Oral contraceptives, clotting factors and thrombosis. *Am J Obstet Gynecol* 142;758–761, 1982

Miller E, Hare JW, Cloherty JP, Dunn PH, Gleason RE, Soeldner JS, Kitzmiller JL: Elevated maternal hemoglobin A1c in early pregnancy and major congenital anomalies in infants of diabetic mothers. *N Engl J Med* 304:1331–1334, 1981

Skouby SO, Anderson O, Saurbrey N, et al.: Oral contraception and insulin sensitivity: in vivo assessment in normal women and women with previous gestational diabetes. *J Clin Endocrinol Metab* 64:519–523, 1987

Skouby SO, Molsted-Pedersen L, Kosonen A: Consequences of intrauterine contraception in diabetic women. *Fert Steril* 42:568–572, 1984

Skouby SO, Kuhl C, Molsted-Pedersen, et al.: Triphasic oral contraception: metabolic effects in normal women and those with previous gestational diabetes. *Am J Obstet Gynecol* 153:495–500, 1985

Speroff L, DeCherney A: Evaluation of a new generation of oral contraceptives. The Advisory Board of the New Progestins. *Obstet Gynecol* 81:1034–1047, 1993

Trussell J: Contraceptive efficacy. In *Contraceptive Technology*. 19th ed. Hatcher RA, Ed. New York, NY, Ardent Media, 2008, p. 19–41

U.S. Medical Eligibility Criteria for Contraceptive Use, 2010. *MMWR* 59:1–85, 2010. Accessed 28 May 2010

Vicente L, Mendonca D, Dingle M, Duarte R, Boavida JM: Etonogestrel implant in women with diabetes mellitus. *Europ J Contracep Repro Health Care* 13:387–395, 2008

Wiese J: Intrauterine contraception in diabetic women. *Fert Steril* 28:422–425, 1977

Wilson ES, Cruickshank J, McMaster M, et al.: A prospective controlled study of the effect on blood pressure of contraceptive preparations containing different types of dosages and progestogen. *Br J Obstet Gynaecol* 91:1254–1260, 1984

Xiang AH, Kawakubo M, Kjos SL, Buchanan TA: Long-acting injectable progestin contraception and risk of type 2 diabetes in Latino women with prior gestational diabetes mellitus. *Diabetes Care* 29:613–617, 2006

# Psychological Impact of Diabetes and Pregnancy

# Highlights
## Psychological Impact of Diabetes and Pregnancy

■ All women go through adjustment stages during their pregnancy, but these are magnified by the diabetes response to the pregnant state.

■ The emotional impact of being pregnant and managing diabetes increases stress levels.

■ Open communication between patient and clinician requires mutual respect, honesty, and cooperation. Open-ended questions provide more information. Condemning nonadherence will not lead to discovering reasons for it.

■ The woman is the final decision maker in handling her day-to-day management. Get her involved to the best of her ability in problem solving and decision making.

■ A psychosocial assessment can provide valuable information about the patient's lifestyle, family, job, and economic situation. This can assist in the development of an individualized care plan to enhance adherence.

■ Emotional support is essential for the patient's well-being, whatever the source—spouse, other family members, health-care professionals, peers, or support groups.

■ Patients with type 1 diabetes (T1D) have an increased awareness of complications. Patients with type 2 diabetes (T2D) often focus concern on whether they will have to continue on insulin after delivery.

■ Concern about having a normal, healthy child or neonatal morbidity is magnified for the pregnant woman with diabetes.

■ High anxiety and fear affect adherence to the pregnancy regimen for tight blood glucose control and dietary adherence. Discussion is essential to assist the patient.

■ Fear tactics do not always improve patient adherence as much as they increase denial and communications breakdown. The intensity of following a strict protocol emotionally lengthens the pregnancy time span for even the most cooperative patient.

■ Prepregnancy counseling is vital for any woman with diabetes of childbearing age, beginning in adolescence.

# Psychological Impact of Diabetes and Pregnancy

Pregnancy is a time of physical and emotional fluctuation for any woman. What is true for any woman, however, becomes intensified for a woman with diabetes, who is faced with increasing demands and scrutiny regarding fetal development, managing her diabetes as it responds to the pregnancy, and increased medical management. Experienced clinicians are aware of how the emotional impact of being pregnant coupled with managing diabetes can increase stress levels for the patient.

Each woman reacts to the diagnosis of diabetes based on her established habits and family–cultural patterns of managing health, which are determined in part by her personality and learned coping methods. Most women have conflicting emotions regarding their diabetes, and even with a wanted pregnancy, they may feel ambivalent.

A myth has developed in our society that everyone should be delighted by the anticipation of having a child. Unfortunately, this illusion sometimes obscures reality. Pregnancy has several major implications for a woman: Her role must expand from being responsible for just herself and her relationship with her mate to including a totally dependent infant; changing body image, involving discomfort at times; a surrender of some amount of her personal freedom for an unspecified period of time; and a commitment of 18–20 years to raising and providing for a child.

When this myth about pregnancy meets reality, a woman's thinking can change as she begins to confront the commitment she is expected to make. Some women feel guilty for having negative feelings they believe are inappropriate. Assurance from her health-care professionals that such feelings are not unusual can be comforting to a woman. Her physician needs to judge whether poor blood glucose control and nonadherence are signals of ambivalence about the pregnancy or a desire to abort or miscarry. It is important not to lose sight of the fact that the only thing all people with diabetes have in common is an elevated blood glucose level.

## RESPONSE TO PREGNANCY IN WOMEN WITH PREEXISTING DIABETES

Most people with diabetes live with some degree of anxiety about their disease, which they deal with in various ways: denial, rationalization, intellectualization, compulsive control, depression, and existential or fatalistic attitude. For a woman with diabetes who becomes pregnant, the natural anxieties related to having diabetes can intensify depending on how well educated she is about her diabetes and what she has been told about bearing and raising children. Furthermore, the increased demands of the complex behavioral regimens utilized during pregnancy can represent a significant obstacle for many women. Evidence regarding strategies that are likely to improve the pregnancy experience for women with diabetes is limited. A small exploratory study in women with pregestational diabetes found that the need to relinquish personal control to health-care professionals and the perception that their diabetes overshadowed the pregnancy were common feelings expressed by the women (Lavender 2010).

She may see her role of child-bearer as a way to prove her self-worth and femininity and her ability to produce a healthy, normal child. These attitudes may increase in importance if she feels some degree of depression related to having diabetes or if she has experienced a previous miscarriage or fetal demise. If the pregnancy is unwanted, negative feelings become intensified, and the potential for residual guilt along with relief increases if the pregnancy is lost, particularly when medical advice has not been followed. In addition, if the advice is that a miscarriage may occur if intensified self-care is not undertaken, then a woman who does not want the pregnancy may use this advice to fulfill a wish to have an abortion.

In the past, it was not unusual for a woman with diabetes to have been told never to bear a child. This misinformation usually was given by a health-care professional who was not aware of the advances in the management of diabetic pregnancy. A woman who has been so misinformed will have increased concern about her risk of developing complications and fears that she may not live long enough to raise her child. In a survey of preconception counseling of 69 women with diabetes, 18 were multiparous, and a large proportion of the women (85%) reported that they knew that their diabetes could affect the health of the baby and good diabetic control was important at the time of conception. The diabetic clinic staff provided ~60% of the advice on preconception glucose control, whereas the other advice came from leaflets or pamphlets. Only 4.5% reported that they heard the advice from "diabetes associations" (Rao 2002). In another study (Diabetes and Pregnancy Group 2005), knowledge about preconception care in French women with type 1 diabetes (T1D) was assessed. Data for all women with T1D in 11 diabetes centers were included. An anonymous dual questionnaire was administered. A total of 138 women were included. The main source of advice about preconception care was noted to be from the physician, and 42% responded that they obtained the advice from a pamphlet. However, 48% claimed that they were unaware of the risk of congenital anomalies related to their blood glucose control, and 41% feared that their baby would be born with diabetes manifesting in the neonatal period. Thus, despite admitting that advice was given about preconception glucose control, the majority of women with T1D have a major knowledge deficit concerning the risks associated with pregnancy. The observation that health-care providers have not been successful in preconception education is at least a first step to solving the problem (Diabetes and Pregnancy Group 2005, Charron-Prochownik 2008).

Because maintaining normal blood glucose levels before becoming pregnant lowers the risk of birth anomalies, make this reassuring information available to patients of childbearing age. Pregnant patients should understand that blood glucose levels can fluctuate regardless of complete adherence to the protocol. In addition, the myth that increased insulin dosages equal worsening diabetes needs to be dismissed: Increased insulin dosage is expected as the placenta grows, and as a result, insulin resistance increases. Patients with type 2 diabetes (T2D) whose prepregnancy diabetes is controlled without insulin but who require insulin injections for normal blood glucose control during pregnancy may be concerned about whether they will remain on insulin after delivery (Rao 2002, Diabetes and Pregnancy Group 2005, Hofmanova 2006).

## RESPONSE TO THE DIAGNOSIS OF GESTATIONAL DIABETES

Nutritional counseling is a priority for the woman with gestational diabetes mellitus. Her education should include information about what gestational diabetes is and why it can occur in pregnancy, the reason for frequent blood testing, and the possibility that insulin may be required later in the pregnancy.

Women with gestational diabetes not only are coping emotionally with the pregnancy but also are confronted with a potentially serious health problem that will become intensified if they are placed on an insulin regimen. The natural anxieties of pregnancy and the fear that they will have to remain on insulin after delivery increase. These fears can affect the ability of the woman with gestational diabetes to learn the necessary daily fundamentals of diabetes management. Personal and cultural health beliefs about diabetes, taking insulin, and why this disease occurred also can affect her ability to learn. Reinforcement and repetition of information are important. The need for repetition, however, is not necessarily a sign of an inherent problem in learning self-care. It is not unusual for an anxious patient to retain only one-third of what originally is taught about diabetes care due to blocking. Some women with gestational diabetes also feel increased ambivalence toward the developing baby. If the diabetes continues after delivery, hostility toward the child, who might be seen as the cause of the diabetes, may be provoked. Being diagnosed and living with gestational diabetes mellitus is a process with both positive and negative dimensions. The majority of women gradually will adapt to the diagnosis and to necessary lifestyle changes with their inconveniences, however, because of their desire for a healthy baby and successful outcome (Persson 2010).

## LONG-TERM ADAPTATION

It is generally difficult to convince anyone that current behavioral changes are important for their continued long-term well-being. Human nature tends to resist change, and when it is required, people look for short-term success. However, permanent behavioral change is not possible unless the individual experiences an attitudinal shift within herself to make the commitment to change her behavior. Even then, permanent behavioral change can take from 6 months to 2 years.

Adapting to the demands of diabetes means changes in lifestyle and daily choices. Diabetes affects spontaneity and relationships with significant others in regard to eating habits, exercise, and self-care. Proper diabetes care takes extra time, thought, preplanning, and other things not usually considered by the nondiabetic person. How well a woman adjusts is affected by prior life experiences and present occurrences in her life as well as her personality, family support (or lack of it), and ways of coping with stress and crisis.

Diabetes self-management education walks a fine line between hope and reality. It is important to support a positive perspective by trying to encourage patients to "slot" the diabetes as just one facet of their life, not the be-all and the end-all. Making a priority list can help point out that life is more than diabetes and that "healthy denial" is valuable because it enables a person with diabetes to cope in a realistic way rather than be burdened with anxiety and depression.

Marked fluctuations in blood glucose levels affect mental and emotional states. It is not much of a quantum jump for some people to fear that diabetes is driving them crazy, particularly if they do not suspect the interrelationship between physiological and psychological body chemistry that research is revealing. Although some degree of mild depression and anxiety is not unusual in diabetes due to its chronicity and potential long-term complications, it need not be uppermost in a person's mind.

An important motivating factor for a pregnant woman with diabetes is remaining healthy to raise her child. The health-care professional's approach is a vital guide in structuring a patient's emotional perspective about herself and her diabetes. The diabetes lifestyle is healthy for everyone. If she can make the commitment to live as balanced a life as possible within the requirements the diabetes establishes, her reward will be feeling healthy and well balanced rather than plagued by illness, fatigue, anxiety, and depression.

## PERSONALITY TYPES AND INDIVIDUALIZING TREATMENT

Numerous studies have revealed that no typical diabetic personality exists (Dunn 1981). Individuals with various personality types make up the population of individuals with diabetes, each with different maturity and intelligence levels and established patterns of coping with the complexities of diabetes and, in this instance, pregnancy.

It is essential to individualize treatment as much as possible to enable the patient to maximize adaptation to a diabetic pregnancy. Taking a psychosocial history is a good first step. Patients are human beings first; having diabetes does not create perfection, although some health-care professionals expect it.

Yet another diabetes myth fostered by clinicians is that, if the patient follows her diabetes treatment plan, her body will respond appropriately. Realistically, diabetes does not always respond to current treatment methodologies. Not only are there many causes for fluctuating blood glucose levels, but patients differ in the level of interest in their condition and treatment as well as capacity for understanding diabetes and accepting and applying information. By becoming sensitive to the variations in patients' needs at different stages in their pregnancy, the clinician becomes more effective in enhancing patient adaptation to the diabetes regimen (Kahana 1964).

The following personality definitions describe the possible psychological profiles a clinician may find in the practice setting, with recommendations for management.

## COMPULSIVE PERSON

*Attitude:* This patient is orderly, controlled with management, and knowledgeable about diabetes and its effects on the body and appears self-disciplined; her driving motivation is related to underlying anxiety of having diabetes.

*Response to management:* This patient is cooperative when treated as an equal; her anxiety level increases when the diabetes does not respond to "perfect" care, with anger toward clinicians if their management is not as rigid as hers. Hospitalization may be difficult because of her having to surrender her independence.

*Management approach:* Make her an active team member with care, decision making, and options; support active participation in self-care; keep her well informed, with discussion and clear communication; give her reassurances that diabetes in pregnancy functions differently than in a nonpregnant state.

## IMMATURE PERSON

*Attitude:* This patient's attitude is inconsistent with management. She exhibits strong denial (disavowing the diabetes), rebellion, anger, resentment, regressive behavior to a younger age level, and childishness.

*Response to management:* This patient has difficulty adhering to the regimen and regularity; dietary indiscretion is common, as is failure to keep appointments and records, refusal to alter lifestyle to any significant degree, hostility toward health-care providers, and potential for a reactive depression if denial is dismantled.

*Management approach:* Use a firm, supportive, nonpunitive manner; use patience; help her recognize that the ability to have the control to make decisions is beneficial to her and her baby. Notice and encourage any positive effort, no matter how small, to follow the regimen; avoid being overly criticial. Comment on dissatisfaction with her behavior and not with her as a person.

## HYSTERICAL PERSON

*Attitude:* This patient is dramatic, emotional, overanxious, and fearful and exhibits strong feelings of being defective secondary to having diabetes.

*Response to management:* This patient watches for the clinician's level of involvement with her case, fears rejection, and worries about regimen and procedures.

*Management approach:* Be consistent and firm, and give continuing reassurance about interest in her case. Focus on her capacity to help herself and what she can do (to help relieve some anxiety and fear).

## DEMANDING DEPENDENT PERSON

*Attitude:* This patient has difficulty with self-management when not pregnant, expects others to care for her diabetes, is petulant and helpless, demands attention, and has deep-seated dependency needs that are not being met.

*Response to management:* This patient wants to be taken care of and have others make all decisions, resists taking responsibility, and seeks extra attention.

*Management approach:* Set reasonable limits within the support offered, communicate and demonstrate interest in her well-being with attention to detail, make telephone contact and extra appointments available if deemed necessary, and praise her for any responsible effort. Cooperation may improve if care is shared by her mate or other family member.

## MASOCHISTIC PERSON

*Attitude:* This patient has a low self-image and diminished self-esteem; she feels she deserves bad luck and may have chronic depression.

*Response to management:* This patient expects misfortune and things to go wrong and may have difficulty following through with the regimen on her own behalf. Depression may limit her ability to learn and apply what is taught; she may chronically complain despite adequate treatment.

*Management approach:* Give consistent support, suggest she follow the regimen for her baby or others if she is unable to do it for herself, show continued interest, and give reassurance and encouragement.

## PASSIVE DEPENDENT PERSON

*Attitude:* This patient wants others to make decisions for her, lacks self-worth, has difficulty making decisions, yields to others' choices, and is submissive.

*Response to management:* She resists taking responsibility or decision making so she cannot be blamed if things do not work, relies on others for support, and may have difficulty acting on recommendations.

*Management approach:* Provide continued support and telephone contact when appointments are not kept and ongoing encouragement and recognition for any efforts with her regimen; enlist help from any support source—mate, family, friends, or agency.

In a study of 100 patients, psychiatric risk factors in diabetic pregnancy were revealed as follows: adolescent pregnancy; previous psychiatric treatment; marital problems; single parenthood; concurrent medical illness (other than diabetes); a history of two or more spontaneous abortions or stillbirths; age >35 years; obesity;

and low socioeconomic status (Barglow 1981). All these factors were overrepresented in women with psychological disturbance.

## DEALING WITH CRISES

### HOSPITALIZATION

Being admitted to the hospital can increase the stress levels for the pregnant woman with diabetes unless she can view it as an acceptable escape from a difficult situation. Some clinicians realize that hospitalization for blood glucose control is not always realistic or desirable, because the patient is no longer functioning in a normal environment, and the separation from her family may create an additional strain.

With the availability of self-monitoring of blood glucose (SMBG) and a team approach providing support and encouragement, many patients develop an enhanced sense of self-control when managing the situation in their own environment. The informed, motivated patient may demonstrate ambivalence during a prolonged hospital stay if she is feeling well and becoming restless and bored by the limited activity. She may resent others making decisions about her health management, particularly if she is excluded from discussions, removed from self-responsibility, and not allowed to share her opinion when she has been able to manage her regimen well at home.

Appropriate dayroom or patio privileges, exercise, and involving the patient in treatment discussions should be allowed to help maintain a balance in her life. The more dependent, less mature patient may enjoy the additional attention she receives during a hospitalization and be quite willing for the staff to take over her diabetes care. She needs limits and encouragement to participate in her management when it is feasible.

### FETAL DEMISE

Most women at some point in their pregnancy have some awareness of the possibility of a fetal loss. This anxiety is particularly intensified in the patient with diabetes. For the woman who very much wants a child, such awareness can increase her anxiety and fear of something happening to her baby. Ordinarily, such anxiety in nondiabetic women is suppressed and superseded by the anticipation of a healthy child.

A woman's response to a fetal loss is determined by several factors: her sociocultural–religious beliefs, the strength of her commitment to have a child, her personality, and her coping capacities in handling loss. There is a psychological as well as physical sense of loss because the experience reinforces her feelings of a lack of normalcy, further damaging her self-image and feminine self-esteem. The anxiety and fear level, already present to some degree, now becomes grounded in reality because her primary feminine function, to produce a healthy child, has been undermined, and she perceives herself as having failed in that role. She not only is threatened by this complication but also is fearful of her capacity to reproduce. Expressions of guilt from not having done certain things related to the regimen dictated by the diabetes are not unusual. If she has followed the regimen to the best of her ability, she can be bitter and angry because she feels the effort she made and the limitations she endured did not matter.

Grieving is a natural and necessary reaction to all types of loss. It enables a person to recognize the finality of the loss and to integrate feelings and thoughts in a healthy way. Increased anxiety is generated by a loss of control over one's life functioning. A fear of potential rejection and abandonment by her partner may exist. Some women become depressed because of anger that has turned inward and that is generated by self-blame, rejection of the imperfect self, and loss of the illusion of invulnerability and omnipotence. This depression is not an unnatural response; the woman has been frustrated and deprived of her goal to have a healthy child. Her depression is a reflection of a realistically unpleasant event that led to an understandable sadness. The symptoms of her sadness may not be consistent and may demonstrate a wavelike quality that increases or recedes at different times.

At such a time, the support of health-care professionals as empathetic listeners should not be underestimated. This healing dimension provides a supportive baseline to the patient with her own healing by providing a sense of participation in living and managing the grieving process. Facilitating the grieving process represents a vital part of caring. It encompasses one's simple presence and availability as a nonjudgmental, receptive listener who accepts and legitimizes the woman's right to her emotions while providing an avenue for their expression when she is ready to do so. Effective management encourages the woman to face her fears and anxiety about a future pregnancy. The expression of such feelings not only assists with her grieving and diminishes denial but also can help her learn to handle any sense of helplessness or hopelessness. The relationship should be maintained at a level that enables her to talk freely and express any feelings.

It is of value to discern the emotional health of the patient and how it relates to her needs. This assessment can be determined not only from the patient but also from her family, other staff members, and her history. It is beneficial to be cognizant of her religious beliefs regarding treatment, family situation, and support system (or lack of it). This awareness can enable the clinician to initiate interventions to assist the patient and her family in meeting their needs. Another consideration may be to share information regarding the prospect of a future pregnancy or possible adoption.

## CONGENITAL ANOMALIES

The woman who delivers an infant with a congenital anomaly may have feelings similar to the patient experiencing a fetal loss or stillbirth. The distinct difference is being confronted with having a child with medical problems, which creates a sense of shock and disbelief. Although the risk of delivering a child with medical problems is known, most people tend to believe that such things happen only to others. The feelings involved with delivering such a baby may last from a few days to years. On a deeper level, there are feelings of hurt pride, wrongdoing, defectiveness, and diminished self-esteem and self-worth.

These emotions need to be handled in a supportive and noncritical manner to enhance healthy self-esteem and encourage a positive attitude for handling the child's condition in a realistic way. It is important to observe and encourage bonding between the mother and her infant. For the most effective bonding to occur, she should be allowed to touch and be with her baby even if the infant is critically ill. Studies have shown that mothers of critically ill or stillborn infants resolve their grieving more rapidly when given the opportunity to be with and hold their baby (Haas 2003). She eventually will require referral to community agencies that can assist and provide services for her and her child.

## THE IMPORTANCE OF A TEAM APPROACH

With rapidly expanding medical technology and knowledge, health-care specialization is increasing, often at the cost of diminished human interaction between health-care professionals and their patients. Because of the complexity of diabetes, a patient can be involved with numerous clinicians. Effective interdisciplinary communication enhances the collaborative effort on the patient's behalf for a successful pregnancy outcome (Wilson 2009).

The patient is the final decision maker in following the advice given and needs to be included whenever feasible in planning her diabetes and pregnancy care. If a problem exists for her in doing so, workable solutions should be implemented after exploring her particular needs. Any discussion with the pregnant patient should encompass the unique role and responsibilities she will have in the management of her pregnancy that differ from the traditional model of the physician having the full responsibility (Anderson 2010). Such an approach can help a woman feel more in control of her daily life, which decreases the potential for hospitalization.

Group discussions and one-on-one counseling with a clinical social worker or psychologist and other patients can provide emotional support and psychosocial problem interventions. It also affords the patient an opportunity for attitudinal change and maturational growth regarding her beliefs about health care, her own maternal and feminine roles, coping options, and herself.

Pregnancy can provide an ideal opportunity for teaching aimed at motivating the patient in improved long-term diabetes management. Educational information can be provided verbally, and printed materials and audiovisual formats are available on diabetes and pregnancy, exercise, breast-feeding, childbirth, sterilization, birth control, postpartum care, and parenting.

Many patients find that, if they are given the responsibility as an equal participant in their care, it is a new health-care management approach for them. In light of prior experiences, it is not unusual for them to be somewhat doubtful initially that they can take this responsibility until they actually see the clinician using such a concept. Even with difficult-to-manage patients, a positive attitudinal effect can result if they are made to feel in control. Treated as a responsible adult and as the unique individual she is, a patient can respond and adapt to the demanding regimen, even when considerable inconvenience is involved, although the requirements emotionally lengthen the pregnancy time span for even the most cooperative patient.

## THE IMPORTANCE OF A SUPPORT SYSTEM

Medical management support and family, peer, and employer attitudes are all influential in determining how a pregnant woman with diabetes adapts to the diabetes and pregnancy regimen. The woman's motivation is heightened if the pregnancy is desired and planned by both partners and if she receives the necessary support from her mate or significant others. Good interfamilial relationships in existence before the pregnancy usually continue. Any preexisting conflict, however, tends to become intensified as the regimen demands place additional strain on the relationship.

The health-care professionals and family members should encourage the woman to accept help from others rather than acquiescing to the convenience of others. This "positive selfishness" is important for her own well-being and that of her baby, particularly for women who are used to managing everything themselves and who find interdependency difficult to accept. Understanding and cooperation regarding medical appointments by employers can enhance a sense of well-being. Group discussions with other patients help develop camaraderie in sharing mutual experience.

The demanding diabetes and pregnancy regimen, with frequent tests and procedures, can create negative feelings in even the most cooperative patient. When recognized and allowed to be expressed, the frustration, fear, anger, and anxiety may be revealed and stress decreased. The health-care professional should discuss with the patient what she can do to heighten her feelings of control over what is happening to her.

When a patient is underinsured or is without insurance coverage, a discussion about the cost of various tests and procedures should be initiated as the pregnancy progresses. The patient or her family may be reluctant to discuss this subject even though it may be of concern.

## SELECTED READINGS

Berg M, Honkasalo ML: Pregnancy and diabetes—a hermeneutic phenomenological study of women's experiences. *J Psychosom Obstet Gynaecol* 21:39–48, 2000

Berg M, Sparud-Lundin C: Experiences of professional support during pregnancy and childbirth: a qualitative study of women with type 1 diabetes. *BMC Pregnancy Childbirth* 9:27–33, 2009

Collier SA, Mulholland C, Williams J, Mersereau P, Turay K, Prue C: A qualitative study of perceived barriers to management of diabetes among women with a history of diabetes during pregnancy. *J Womens Health* 20:1333–1339, 2011

Daniells S, Grenyer BF, Davis WS, Coleman KJ, Burgess JA, Moses RG: Gestational diabetes mellitus: is a diagnosis associated with an increase in maternal anxiety and stress in the short and intermediate term? *Diabetes Care* 26:385–389, 2003

Katon JG, Russo J, Gavin AR, Melville JL, Katon WJ: Diabetes and depression in pregnancy: is there an association? *J Womens Health* 20:983–989, 2011

Levy-Shiff R, Har-Even D, Lerman M, Hod M: Maternal adjustment and infant outcome in medically defined high-risk pregnancy. *Developmental Psychology* 38:93–103, 2002

Mersereau P, Williams J, Collier SA, Mulholland C, Turay K, Prue C: Barriers to managing diabetes during pregnancy: the perceptions of health care practitioners. *Birth* 38:142–149, 2011

Murphy HR: Integrating educational and technological interventions to improve pregnancy outcomes in women with diabetes. *Diabetes Obes Metab* 12:97–104, 2010

Rasmussen-Torvik LJ, Harlow BL: The association between depression and diabetes in the perinatal period. *Curr Diabetes Rep* 10:217–223, 2010

Rodgers Fischl AF, Herman WH, Sereika SM, Hannan M, Becker D, Mansfield MJ, Freytag LL, Milaszewski K, Botscheller AN, Charron-Prochownik D: Impact of a preconception counseling program for teens with type 1 diabetes (Ready-Girls) on patient-provider interaction, resource utilization and cost. *Diabetes Care* 33:701–705, 2010

Sacks DA: Preconception care for diabetic women: background, barriers, and strategies for effective implementation. *Curr Diabetes Rev* 2:147–161, 2006

Wahabi HA, Alzeidan RA, Bawazeer GA, Alansari LA, Esmaeil SA: Preconception care for diabetic women for improving maternal and fetal outcomes: a systematic review and meta-analysis. *BMC Pregnancy Childbirth* 10:63–77, 2010

---

## REFERENCES

Anderson RM, Funnell MM: Patient empowerment: myths and misconceptions. *Patient Educ Couns* 79:277–282, 2010

Barglow P, Hatcher R, Wolston J, Phelps R, Burns W, Depp R: Psychiatric risk factors in the pregnant diabetic patient. *Am J Obstet Gynecol* 140:46–52, 1981

Charron-Prochownik D, Hannan MF, Fischl AR, Slocum JM: Preconception planning: Are we making progress? *Curr Diabetes Rep* 8:294–298, 2008

Diabetes and Pregnancy Group: Knowledge about preconception care in French women with type 1 diabetes. *Diabetes Metab* 31:443–447, 2005

Dunn SM, Turtle JR: The myth of the diabetic personality. *Diabetes Care* 4:640–46, 1981

Haas F: Bereavement care: seeing the body. *Nursing Standard* 17:33–37, 2003

Hofmanova I: Pre-conception care and support for women with diabetes (Review). *Br J Nurs* 15:90–94, 2006

Kahana R, Bibring D: Personality types in medical management. In *Psychiatry and Medical Practice in a General Hospital.* Zinberg NE, Ed. New York, International University Press, 1964, p. 108–123

Lavender T, Platt MJ, Tsekiri E, Casson I, Byrom S, Baker L, Walkinshaw S: Women's perceptions of being pregnant and having pregestational diabetes. *Midwifery* 26:589–595, 2010

Persson M, Winkvist A, Mogren I: "From stun to gradual balance"—women's experiences of living with gestational diabetes mellitus. *Scand J Caring Sci* 24:454–462, 2010

Rao S, Lindow SW, Masson EA: Survey of pre-conception counseling. *Diabet Med* 19:615, 2002

Wilson N, Ashawesh K, Kulambil Padinjakara RN, Anwar A: The multidisciplinary diabetes-endocrinology clinic and postprandial blood glucose monitoring in the management of gestational diabetes: impact on maternal and neonatal outcomes. *Exp Clin Endocrinol Diabetes* 117:486–489, 2009

# Assessment of Glycemic Control

# Highlights
## Assessment of Glycemic Control

■ Hyperglycemia is the major cause of complications of diabetes and pregnancy.

■ Normoglycemia minimizes these complications.

■ Continued attention to blood glucose control is mandatory on the part of the woman and her health-care team.

# Assessment of Glycemic Control

## NORMOGLYCEMIA DURING PREGNANCY

Studies of intermittent capillary blood glucose and continuous interstitial glucose monitoring in normal pregnant women in their usual settings revealed a rather narrow range of glucose concentrations. Fasting plasma glucose concentrations decline modestly, by ~2 mg/dl, in early normal pregnancy (Mills 1998). There is a slight, gradual rise in mean and postprandial glucose values throughout the second and third trimesters of normal pregnancy. In nondiabetic pregnant women, reference ranges for capillary fasting, overnight, and premeal glucose calibrated to plasma levels are 50–99 mg/dl, with postmeal peak values 60–70 min after eating of 81–129 mg/dl (Table 4.1) (Parretti 2001, Yogev 2004).

## SELF-MONITORING OF CAPILLARY BLOOD GLUCOSE

Self-monitoring of blood glucose (SMBG) is an integral part of the intensified treatment of diabetes that has dramatically improved pregnancy outcome over the past 25 years (Sacks 2002, American Diabetes Association 2011) and is necessary for individuals to achieve optimal glucose goals. Capillary blood glucose refers to the usual sample obtained by the patient; it is recognized that most glucose meters now calibrate capillary blood measurements to read as plasma glucose for comparability with reference laboratory measurements; hence, in this chapter, the use of SMBG implies that fact. The amount of glucose per unit water mass is the same in whole blood and plasma. According to Sacks (2002), "Although red blood cells are essentially freely permeable to glucose (glucose is taken up by facilitated transport), the concentration of water in plasma (kg/l) is ~11% higher than that of whole blood. Therefore, glucose concentrations in plasma are ~11% higher than whole blood if the hematocrit is normal."

Because this is true for glucose values measured in venous or capillary blood (Chmielewski 1995; International Federation of Clinical Chemistry and Laboratory Medicine, Scientific Division Working Group on Selective Electrodes, 2001; Kuwa 2001; Torjman 2001; Buhling 2003), "it is crucial that people with diabetes know whether their monitor and strips provide whole blood or plasma results" (American Diabetes Association 2011). The National Academy of Clinical Biochemistry's guideline for management of diabetes adopted by the American Diabetes Association (Sacks 2002), however, has suggested that the total error of meter use (user plus analytical) is often as much as the difference between whole blood and plasma glucose measurement, as noted by others (Parkes 2000, Boehme

**Table 4.1 Normal Glucose Concentrations (mg/dl) and A1C Levels during Third Trimester of Pregnancy, Capillary Glucose and A1C Goals for Women with Preexisting Diabetes before and during Early Pregnancy, and Optimal Goals during the Second and Third Trimesters**

| Group | Daily mean glucose | Fasting, premeal, nighttime | 1-h post-prandial | 2-h post-prandial | A1C (%) |
|---|---|---|---|---|---|
| Normal pregnancy (mean and SD) | | | | | 4.8 (0.4)** |
| Capillary glucose by meter* (Paretti 2001) | 82.9 ± 5.8 | 69.3 ± 5.7 | 108.4 ± 6 | | |
| Continuous interstitial glucose (Yogev 2004) | 83.7 ± 18 | 76.6 ± 11.5 | 105.3 ± 12 | 97.2 ± 10 | |
| Goals during the second and third trimesters | <110*** | 60-99*** | <140**** | <120**** | <6.0*** |

*Adjusted to be equivalent to plasma glucose values.

**From Lowe LP, Metzger BE, Dyer AR, et al., for the HAPO Study Cooperative Research Group: Hyperglycemia and Adverse Pregnancy Outcome (HAPO) study: associations of maternal A1C and glucose with pregnancy outcomes. *Diabetes Care* 35:574–580, 2012

***From Kitzmiller JL, Block JM, Brown FM, et al.: ADA consensus statement: managing preexisting diabetes for pregnancy. *Diabetes Care* 31:1060–1079, 2008

****From American College of Obstetricians and Gynecologists: Pregestational diabetes mellitus. ACOG Practice Bulletin No. 60. *Obstet Gynecol* 105:675–685, 2005 (reaffirmed 2010)

2003). The higher the glucose value, the greater the variance of capillary glucose measurements compared with a reference plasma method seems to be (Boehme 2003). In studies of the accuracy of SMBG in the normo- to hyperglycemic range in pregnant women with diabetes, usage of most home devices had a total error of <15% (Moses 1997, Henry 2001). In the hypoglycemic range, there may be a reduction in the accuracy of SMBG (Moberg 1993, Zenobi 1995, Trajanoski 1996), perhaps because of alterations in subcutaneous blood flow during hypoglycemia (Hilsted 1985, Fernqvist-Forbes 1988, Aman 1992).

SMBG allows the patient to evaluate her individual response to therapy and assess whether glycemic targets are being achieved. Frequent sampling is optimal in pregnancy because of the increased potential for rapid-onset hypoglycemia in the absence of food or presence of exercise and the exacerbated hyperglycemic responses to food ingestion, psychological stress, and intercurrent illness related to gestational insulin resistance. Use of glucose meters with memory capacity is important for verification of the reliability of patient self-testing and recording (Langer 1986). The accuracy of SMBG is instrument and user dependent (Sacks 2002), and it is important for health-care providers to evaluate each patient's SMBG technique, both initially and at regular intervals thereafter. The patient should "use calibrators and controls on a regular basis to assure accuracy of results" (American Diabetes Association 2011). Optimal use of SMBG requires proper interpretation of the data, and many patients can be taught how to use the data to adjust food intake, exercise, or insulin therapy to achieve specific glycemic goals. Health-care professionals regularly should evaluate the patient's ability to use data to guide therapy.

## SITE OF SMBG

To provide less painful glucose self-testing, manufacturers developed products designed for use at alternative sites—usually the forearm or thigh (American Diabetes Association 2011). When glucose concentrations are rapidly rising or falling (e.g., postprandially, immediately after exercise, or with insulin-induced hypoglycemia), however, there is a lag time between the fingerstick capillary glucose concentration and the alternative site testing of the forearm and thigh (Ellison 2002, Jungheim 2002, Bina 2003). Therefore, use of alternative site testing systems in the dynamic state of pregnancy will give different results than fingerstick testing (American Diabetes Association 2011) and is not wise. Palm and fingertip capillary glucose values are similar at different time points (Bina 2003, Meguro 2005), but these testing sites have not been compared in pregnancy.

## TIMING OF SMBG

A randomized trial of premeal versus postprandial glucose testing as the guide for insulin therapy in pregnant women with gestational diabetes mellitus (GDM) severe enough to require treatment beyond diet reported lower frequencies of perinatal complications with the treatment strategy based on postmeal testing (de Veciana 1995). A similar result was found in a randomized trial of premeal versus postprandial testing starting at 16 weeks of gestation in women with type 1 diabetes (T1D) (Manderson 2003). These trials support the previous observational studies in T1D and type 2 diabetes (T2D) that revealed postprandial glucose levels as the best predictor of fetal macrosomia (Jovanovic 1991, Combs 1992, Parretti 2003). Because most pregnant patients with T1D or T2D will use short-acting insulin injections before meals to prevent postprandial hyperglycemia, additional premeal glucose testing may be useful to allow temporary adjustments of insulin dose if the glucose level is low or elevated (Skyler 1981, Hirsch 1998). Bedtime and overnight blood glucose testing is used as needed to detect hyper- or hypoglycemia at those time points to allow subsequent adjustment of snacks or insulin doses.

The protocols for the timing and frequency of self-monitored glucose concentrations should be designed to reflect the peak and the nadir of maternal glycemia. Previously when animal regular insulin was prescribed, and even with the advent of recombinant DNA technology that made available human regular insulin, the concern that the peak action of the regular insulin might cause hypoglycemic reactions 1.5–2.5 h after the injection led to usage of the 2-h postprandial time point. Because the available rapid-acting insulin analogs have peak effect at 45–70 min after injection, and because the concern is to prevent hyperglycemia-induced fetal complications, 1-h postprandial testing may be better in pregnancies complicated by diabetes. Studies with continuous interstitial glucose monitoring in pregnant women with diabetes show the mean peak postprandial glucose to average 90 min after beginning the meal, with considerable variation from patient to patient (Ben-Haroush 2004) and high day-to-day variability (Kerssen 2004a). Teaching patients to test at 1 h after beginning the meal should approximate these peaks. Some pregnant patients may have delayed postprandial peak glucose excursions related to delayed gastric emptying (Stanley 1995). It also is recognized that meals with high fat content in pregnancy may prolong the postprandial glucose excursion. A study in which 68 women with GDM used SMBG at both 1 and 2 h postprandial for 1 week after diagnosis revealed a greater proportion of abnormal values at 1 h after breakfast and equivalence after lunch, but a greater proportion of abnormal values at 2 h after dinner (Sivan 2001). Either 1-h or 2-h testing is acceptable.

Continuous glucose monitoring (CGM) devices measure subcutaneous interstitial tissue glucose by an electrochemical method. Because interstitial fluid glucose levels are 20–50% lower than blood glucose levels (Rebrin 1999), calibration with several capillary glucose levels per day corrects for this difference (Kerssen 2006). Feasibility studies of older CGM systems in pregnancies of women with T1D treated with multiple daily insulin injections revealed periods of both hyper- and hypoglycemia that were not detected by fingerstick testing or patient symptoms (Yogev 2003a, 2003b; Ben-Haroush 2004; Kerssen 2004b, 2006). Interstitial glucose values failed to reflect symptomatic hypoglycemia confirmed by capillary glucose testing in 6.2% of all paired samples in a study of 15 pregnant women with T1D (Kerssen 2006), and reproducibility of glucose measurements in subjects wearing two sensors at the same time is not optimal (Metzger 2002, Guerci 2003, Larsen 2004). CGM devices provide real-time glucose data to patients and have alarms for both glucose values out of range and for rapidly changing glucose values. To make treatment decisions (such as calculating premeal insulin doses), however, patients are advised to use SMBG values. Prospective controlled trials are needed to determine whether application of this expensive method to fine-tune glycemic control will improve perinatal outcome and maternal safety. Ancillary questions include which patients might benefit the most and at which stages of pregnancy.

## OTHER MEASURES OF METABOLIC CONTROL

Glycated hemoglobin (GHb) is the general term used to describe a series of stable minor hemoglobin components formed slowly and nonenzymatically in direct proportion to the ambient glucose concentration (Sacks 2002, American Diabetes Association 2011). GHb values expressed as the percentage of total hemoglobin provide the best assessment of the degree of chronic glycemic control, reflecting the average blood glucose concentration during the preceding 6–12 weeks because the life span of the red blood cells is shortened to <90 days in pregnancy (Lurie 1992). GHb can be misleading if patients balance frequent low and high blood glucose levels, however, because this indicator of average glucose would not reflect postprandial elevations, which could represent important pulses of high glucose in the fetus (Derr 2003, Kerssen 2007). Many GHb assays are available, but A1C has become the preferred standard for assessing glycemic control (Sacks 2002, American Diabetes Association 2011). When maternal glycemia is elevated and rapidly brought toward normal in pregnancy, A1C has been reported to show a significant decrease within 2 weeks compared with the baseline elevation. Thus, the measurement of A1C every 2–4 weeks confirms the SMBG measurements. Standardization of laboratory A1C measurements has been achieved by the vast majority of U.S. laboratories (Marshall 2000; Sacks 2002, 2005; American Diabetes Association 2011), because a variety of reference limits have been obtained with different high-performance liquid chromatography (HPLC) equipment (Parentoni 1998). Manufacturers of A1C test methods can earn a certificate of traceability to the Diabetes Control and Complications Trial (DCCT) reference method (Rohlfing 2002) by passing rigorous testing criteria for precision and accuracy (Sacks 2002, American Diabetes Association 2011). One highly sensitive, precise, and accurate HPLC method yielded a reference range (2.5 and 97.5 percentiles) of 3.2–4.3 for 63 healthy pregnant women, compared with 3.4–4.9 in other adult women (Parentonia 1998). Evaluation of DCCT-aligned ion-exchange liquid chromatography assays revealed lower reference ranges for A1C in 493 and 100 healthy pregnant women of 4.1–5.9 and 4.5–5.7, respectively, compared with 4.7–6.3 in age-matched nonpregnant control women (O'Kane 2001, Nielsen 2004). The results were not affected by differences in body mass between groups. Trimester- and ethnic group–related differences in A1C in different stages of normal pregnancy are not of clinical significance (Parentoni 1998, Hartland 1999, O'Kane 2001).

Glycated serum protein assays correlate well with the A1C test (Sacks 2002, American Diabetes Association 2011). Although the measurement of fructosamine, an indirect measurement of glycosylated serum proteins (mostly albumin), theoretically should reflect the average blood glucose over the past week because of the rapid turnover rate of albumin (8 days in pregnancy), fructosamine has not proved to be useful in pregnancies complicated by diabetes. Because fructosamine assays are an indirect measurement of total glycosylated serum proteins, there is interference by reducing agents in the blood. If a pregnant woman recently has taken her prenatal vitamins, then the results of the fructosamine assay will vary based on her blood concentrations of vitamin C. Vitamin C concentrations in the blood alter the fructosamine assay more than small changes in glycemia. In addition, there is a diurnal variation in serum protein concentrations in the blood. Thus, the woman must have her fructosamine test at the same time for each determination or the variation in total serum proteins may be greater than the change in this measure of average blood glucose concentrations.

## KETONURIA AND KETONEMIA

Ketone testing is important, as the presence of ketones can indicate impending diabetic ketoacidosis (DKA), which may develop quickly in pregnancy in women with T1D. Urine ketones should be measured periodically when the pregnant woman with diabetes is ill or when any blood glucose value is >180 mg/dl. Outside pregnancy, 300 mg/dl is used, but a lower threshold is used in pregnancy because DKA can develop at lower levels of hyperglycemia in pregnant women with T1D or T2D (Whiteman 1996, Montoro 2004). DKA is associated with a high mortality rate in the fetus (Montoro 2004). In addition, fasting ketonemia in pregnant diabetic and nondiabetic women has been associated with decreased intelligence and fine motor skills in offspring (Rizzo 1991). Women with moderate to large ketonuria associated with hyperglycemia should alert their physician immediately for a determination of ketonemia and serum electrolytes. Urine ketone tests are not reliable for the firm diagnosis of DKA, which is better made with blood ketone testing that quantifies β-hydroxybutyric acid (Sacks 2002, American Diabetes Association 2011). Home tests for β-hydroxybutyric acid are available, but they have not been evaluated systematically in pregnancy.

## RECOMMENDATIONS

- SMBG is a key component of diabetes therapy during pregnancy in women with T1D, T2D, and GDM and should be included in the management plan. Daily SMBG will provide optimal results in pregnancy.
- Fingerstick SMBG testing is best in pregnancy, as alternative site testing may not identify rapid changes in blood glucose concentrations characteristic of pregnant women with preexisting diabetes.
- Instruct the patient in SMBG using meters with memory capacity, and routinely evaluate the patient's technique and ability to use data to adjust therapy. SMBG as used here implies current glucose meters that calibrate blood glucose readings to plasma glucose values. Ideally, provide the pregnant patient with the opportunity for daily telephone or electronic contact with the health-care staff to discuss problems in management.
- Postprandial capillary glucose measured 1 h after beginning the meal best approximates postmeal peak glucose measured continuously.
- Because of individual differences in time to peak postprandial glucose level related to gastric emptying, content and time of meals, and possibly other factors, it may be optimal for each patient to determine her own peak postprandial glucose testing time after breakfast, lunch, and dinner. Either 1-h or 2-h postmeal testing is an acceptable approach.
- Generally target fasting, overnight, and premeal plasma glucose values of 60–99 mg/dl, 1-h postmeal plasma glucose values of <140 mg/dl, 2-h postmeal values of <120 mg/dl, and mean daily plasma glucose <110 mg/dl to achieve optimal pregnancy outcome.
- SMBG targets should be tailored to individual patient characteristics, such as hypoglycemia unawareness.
- Teach the patient to test capillary plasma glucose appropriately to prevent, identify, and treat hypoglycemia.
- The use of continuous interstitial glucose monitoring needs more evaluation before it can be recommended for general use in pregnant women with diabetes.
- Teach the pregnant patient to perform urine ketone measurements at times of illness or when the blood glucose reaches 180 mg/dl. Positive values should be reported promptly to the health-care professional.
- Perform the A1C test at the initial visit during pregnancy and then monthly until target levels <6.2% in a DCCT-aligned assay are achieved; then every 2–4 months should be sufficient.

## SELECTED READINGS

American College of Obstetricians and Gynecologists: Pregestational diabetes mellitus. ACOG Practice Bulletin No. 60. *Obstet Gynecol* 105:675–685, 2005 (reaffirmed 2010)

American Diabetes Association: Position statement executive summary: tests of glycemia in diabetes. *Diabetes Care* 34 (Suppl. 1):S1419–S1423, 2011

## REFERENCES

Aman J, Berne C, Ewald U, Tuvemo T: Cutaneous blood flow during a hypoglycemic clamp in insulin-dependent diabetic patients and healthy subjects. *Clin Sci* 82:615–618, 1992

American College of Obstetricians and Gynecologists: Pregestational diabetes mellitus. ACOG Practice Bulletin #60, 2005 (reaffirmed 2010). *Obstet Gynecol* 105:675–685, 2005

American Diabetes Association: Position statement executive summary: tests of glycemia in diabetes. *Diabetes Care* 34 (Suppl. 1):S1419–S1423, 2011

Ben-Haroush A, Yogev Y, Chen R, Rosenn B, Hod M, Langer O: The postprandial glucose profile in the diabetic pregnancy. *Am J Obstet Gynecol* 191:576–581, 2004

Bina DM, Anderson RL, Johnson ML, Bergenstal RM, Kendall DM: Clinical impact of prandial state, exercise, and site preparation on the equivalence of alternative-site blood glucose testing. *Diabetes Care* 26:981–985, 2003

Boehme P, Floriot M, Sirveaux M-A, Durain D, Ziegler O, Drouin P, Guerci B: Evolution of analytical performance in portable glucose meters in the last decade. *Diabetes Care* 26:1170–1175, 2003

Buhling KJ, Henrich W, Kjos SL, Siebert G, Starr E, Dreweck C, Stein U, Dudenhausen JW: Comparison of point-of-care-testing glucose meters with standard laboratory measurement of the 50 g-glucose-challenge test (GCT) during pregnancy. *Clin Biochem* 36:333–337, 2003

Chmielewski SA: Advances and strategies for glucose monitoring. *Am J Clin Pathol* 104 (Suppl. 1):S59–S71, 1995

Combs CA, Gunderson E, Kitzmiller JL, Gavin LA, Main EK: Relationship of fetal macrosomia to maternal postprandial glucose control during pregnancy. *Diabetes Care* 15:1251–1257, 1992

Derr R, Garrett E, Stacy GA, Suadek CD: Is HbA1c affected by glycemic instability? *Diabetes Care* 26:2728–2733, 2003

de Veciana M, Major CA, Morgan MA, Asrat T, Toohey JS, Lien JM, Evans AT: Postprandial versus preprandial blood glucose monitoring in women with gestational diabetes mellitus requiring insulin therapy. *N Engl J Med* 333:1237–1241, 1995

Ellison JM, Stegman JM, Colner SL, Michael RH, Sharma MK, Ervin KR, Horwitz DL: Rapid changes in postprandial blood glucose produce concentration differences at finger, forearm, and thigh sampling sites. *Diabetes Care* 25:961–964, 2002

Fernqvist-Forbes E, Linde B, Gunnarsson R: Insulin absorption and subcutaneous blood flow in normal subjects during hypoglycemia in man. *J Clin Endocrinol Metab* 67:619–623, 1988

Guerci B, Floriot M, Bohme P, Durain D, Benichou M, Jellimann S, Drouin P: Clinical performance of CGMS in type 1 diabetic patients treated by continuous subcutaneous glucose insulin infusion using insulin analogs. *Diabetes Care* 26:582–589, 2003

Hartland AJ, Smith JM, Clarke PMS, Webber J, Chowdhury T, Dunne F: Establishing trimester- and ethnic group-related reference ranges for fructosamine and HBA1c in non-diabetic pregnant women. *Ann Clin Biochem* 36:235–237, 1999

Henry MJ, Major CA, Reinsch S: Accuracy of self-monitoring of blood glucose: impact on diabetes management decisions during pregnancy. *Diabetes Educ* 27:521–529, 2001

Hilsted J, Bonde-Petersen F, Madsbad S, Parving HH, Christensen NJ, Adelhoj B, Bigler D, Sjontoft E: Changes in plasma volume, in transcapillary escape rate of albumin and in subcutaneous blood flow during hypoglycemia in man. *Clin Sci* 69:273–277, 1985

Hirsch IB: Intensive treatment of type 1 diabetes. *Med Clin N Am* 82:689–719, 1998

International Federation of Clinical Chemistry and Laboratory Medicine, Scientific Division Working Group on Selective Electrodes: IFCC recommendation on reporting results for blood glucose. *Clin Chim Acta* 307:205–209, 2001

Jovanovic L, Peterson CM, Reed GF, Metzger BE, Mills JL, Knopp RH, Aarons JH: Maternal postprandial glucose levels and infant birth weight: the Diabetes in Early Pregnancy study. The National Institute of Child Health and Human Development—Diabetes in Early Pregnancy Study. *Am J Obstet Gynecol* 164:103–111, 1991

Jungheim K, Koschinsky T: Glucose monitoring in the arm: risky delays of hypoglycemia and hyperglycemia detection. *Diabetes Care* 25:956–960, 2002

Kerssen A, de Valk HW, Visser GH: Increased second trimester maternal glucose levels are related to extreme large-for-gestational age infants in women with type 1 diabetes mellitus. *Diabetes Care* 30:1069–1074, 2007

Kerssen A, de Valk HW, Visser GH: Do HbA1c levels and the self-monitoring of blood glucose levels adequately reflect glycemic control during pregnancy in women with type 1 diabetes mellitus? *Diabetologia* 49:25–28, 2006

Kerssen A, de Valk HW, Visser GHA: Day-to-day glucose variability during pregnancy in women with type 1 diabetes mellitus: glucose profiles measured with the continuous glucose monitoring system. *BJOG* 111:919–924, 2004a

Kerssen A, de valk HW, Visser GHA: The continuous glucose monitoring system during pregnancy of women with type 1 diabetes mellitus: accuracy assessment. *Diabetes Technol Ther* 6:645–651, 2004b

Kitzmiller JL, Block JM, Brown FM, et al.: ADA consensus statement: managing preexisting diabetes for pregnancy. *Diabetes Care* 31:1060–1079, 2008

Kuwa K, Nakayama T, Hoshino T, Tominaga M: Relationships of glucose concentrations in capillary whole blood, venous whole blood and venous plasma. *Clin Chim Acta* 307:187–192, 2001

Langer O, Mazze RS: Diabetes in pregnancy: evaluating self-monitoring performance and glycemic control with memory-based reflectance meters. *Am J Obstet Gynecol* 155:635–637, 1986

Larsen J, Ford T, Lyden E, Colling C, Mack-Shipman L, Lane J: What is hypoglycemia in patients with well-controlled type 1 diabetes treated by subcutaneous insulin pump with use of the continuous glucose monitoring system? *Endocr Pract* 10:324–329, 2004

Lowe LP, Metzger BE, Dyer AR, et al., for the HAPO Study Cooperative Research Group: Hyperglycemia and Adverse Pregnancy Outcome (HAPO) study: associations of maternal A1C and glucose with pregnancy outcomes. *Diabetes Care* 35:574–580, 2012

Lurie S, Danon D: Life span of erythrocytes in late pregnancy. *Obstet Gynecol* 80:123–126, 1992

Manderson JG, Patterson CC, Hadden DR, Traub AI, Ennis C, McCance DR: Preprandial versus postprandial blood glucose monitoring in type 1 diabetic pregnancy: a randomized controlled clinical trial. *Am J Obstet Gynecol* 189:507–512, 2003

Marshall SM, Barth JH: Standardization of HbA1c measurements: a consensus statement. *Diabet Med* 17:5–6, 2000

Meguro S, Funae O, Hosokawa K, Atsumi Y: Hypoglycemia detection rate differs among blood glucose monitoring sites. *Diabetes Care* 28:708–709, 2005

Metzger M, Leibowitz G, Wainstein J, Glaser B, Raz I: Reproducibility of glucose measurements using the glucose sensor. *Diabetes Care* 25:1185–1191, 2002

Mills JL, Jovanovic, L, Knopp R, Aarons J, Conley M, Park E, Lee YJ, Holmes L, Simpson JL, Metzger B: Physiological reduction in fasting blood glucose concentration in the first trimester of normal pregnancy: The Diabetes in Early Pregnancy Study. *Metabolism* 47:1140–1144, 1998

Moberg E, Lundblad S, Lins P-E, Adamson U: How accurate are home blood-glucose meters with special respect to the low glycemic range? *Diabetes Res Clin Pract* 19:239–243, 1993

Montoro MN: Diabetic ketoacidosis in pregnancy. In *Diabetes in Women: Adolescence, Pregnancy, and Menopause.* 3rd ed. Reece EA, Coustan DR, and Gabbe SG, Eds. Philadelphia, PA, Lippincott Williams & Wilkins, 2004, p. 345–350

Moses R, Schier G, Mathews J, Davis W: The accuracy of home glucose meters for the glucose range anticipated in pregnancy. *Aust N Z J Obstet Gynecol* 37:282–286, 1997

Nielsen LR, Ekbom P, Damm P, Glumer C, Frandsen MM, Jensen DM, Mathiesen ER: HbA1c levels are significantly lower in early and late pregnancy. *Diabetes Care* 27:1200–1201, 2004

O'Kane MJ, Lynch PLM, Moles KW, Magee SE: Determination of a Diabetes Control and Complications Trial-aligned HbA1c reference range in pregnancy. *Clin Chim Acta* 311:157–159, 2001

Parentoni LS, de Faria EC, Bartelega MJLF, Moda VMS, Facin ACC, Castilho LN: Glycated hemoglobin reference limits obtained by high performance liquid chromatography in adults and pregnant women. *Clin Chim Acta* 274:105–109, 1998

Parkes JL, Slatin SL, Pardo S, Ginsberg BH: A new consensus error grid to evaluate the clinical significance of inaccuracies in the measurement of blood glucose. *Diabetes Care* 23:1143–1148, 2000

Parretti E, Carignani L, Cioni R, Bartoli E, Borri P, La Torre P, Mecacci F, Martini E, Scarselli G, Mello G: Sonographic evaluation of fetal growth and body composition in women with different degrees of normal glucose metabolism. *Diabetes Care* 26:2741–2748, 2003

Parretti E, Mecaci F, Papini M, Cioni R, Carignani L, Mignosa M, La Torre P, Mello G: Third-trimester maternal blood glucose levels from diurnal profiles in nondiabetic pregnancies: correlation with sonographic parameters of fetal growth. *Diabetes Care* 24:1319–1323, 2001

Rebrin K, Steil GM, van Antwerp WP, Mastrototaro JJ: Subcutaneous glucose predicts plasma glucose independent of insulin: implications for continuous monitoring. *Am J Physiol* 277:E561–E571, 1999

Rizzo T, Metzger BE, Burns WJ, Burns K: Correlations between antepartum maternal metabolism and child intelligence. *N Engl J Med* 325:911–916, 1991

Rohlfing CL, Wiedmeyer HM, Little RR, England JD, Tennill A, Goldstein DE: Defining the relationship between plasma glucose and HbA1c: analysis of glucose profiles and HbA1c in the Diabetes Control and Complications Trial. *Diabetes Care* 25:275–278, 2002

Sacks DB, ADA/EASD/IDF Working Group of the HbA1c Assay: Global harmonization of hemoglobin A1c. *Clin Chem* 51:681–683, 2005

Sacks DB, Arnold M, Bakris GL, Bruns DE, et al.: Guidelines and recommendations for laboratory analysis in the diagnosis and management of diabetes mellitus (Position Statement). *Diabetes Care* 25:750–786, 2002

Sivan E, Weisz B, Homko CJ, Reece EA, Schiff E: One or two hours postprandial glucose measurements: are they the same? *Am J Obstet Gynecol* 185:604–607, 2001

Skyler JS, Skyler DL, Seigler DE, O'Sullivan MJ: Algorithms for adjustment of insulin dosage by patients who monitor blood glucose. *Diabetes Care* 4:311–318, 1981

Stanley K, Magides A, Arnot M, Bruce C, Reilly C, McFee A, Fraser R: Delayed gastric emptying as a factor in delayed postprandial glycemic response in pregnancy. *Brit J Obstet Gynecol* 102:288–291, 1995

Torjman MC, Jahn L, Joseph JI, Crothall K, Goldstein BJ: Accuracy of the HemoCue portable glucose analyzer in a large nonhomogeneous population. *Diabetes Technol Therapeut* 3:591–600, 2001

Trajanoski Z, Brunner GA, Gfrerer RJ, Wach P, Pieber TR: Accuracy of home blood glucose meters during hypoglycemia. *Diabetes Care* 19:1412–1415, 1996

Whiteman VE, Homko CJ, Reece EA: Management of hypoglycemia and diabetic ketoacidosis in pregnancy. *Obstet Gynecol Clinics N Am* 23:87–107, 1996

Yogev Y, Ben-Haroush A, Chen R, Rosenn B, Hod M, Langer O: Diurnal glycemic profile in obese and normal weight nondiabetic pregnant women. *Am J Obstet Gynecol* 191:949–953, 2004

Yogev Y, Ben-Haroush A, Chen R, Kaplan B, Phillip M, Hod M: Continuous glucose monitoring for treatment adjustment in diabetic pregnancies: a pilot study. *Diabet Med* 20:558–562, 2003a

Yogev Y, Chen R, Ben-Haroush A, Phillip M, Jovanovic L, Hod M: Continuous glucose monitoring for the evaluation of gravid women with type 1 diabetes mellitus. *Obstet Gynecol* 101:633–638, 2003b

Zenobi PD, Keller A, Jaeggi-Groisman SE, Glatz Y: Accuracy of devices for self-monitoring of blood glucose including hypoglycemic blood glucose levels. *Diabetes Care* 18:587–588, 1995

# Management of Morning Sickness

# Highlights
## Management of Morning Sickness

■ Patients suffering from morning sickness should eat six small meals each day, avoiding spicy and fatty foods and caffeine.

■ When nausea is a symptom of premeal hypoglycemia, options are to decrease the premeal insulin dose, shorten the insulin-meal interval, or have the patient take a portion of the insulin dose with a meal's carbohydrate to test tolerance to food before the rest of the insulin dose is taken.

■ If vomiting continues for >8 h, hospitalization for fluid replacement may be necessary. If intravenous therapy is required, blood glucose levels should be maintained in the normal range.

# Management of Morning Sickness

Morning sickness—nausea or vomiting during pregnancy—is one of the most common symptoms of early pregnancy, affecting 70–85% of pregnant women (American College of Obstetricians and Gynecologists 2004). It is usually a tolerable annoyance for most women, but if the pregnant woman also has diabetes, the management of morning sickness requires special attention. Although it is termed morning sickness because it occurs most frequently on waking and lessens as the day continues, nausea and vomiting may occur at any time of day and even, on occasion, all day.

The cause of morning sickness is not completely understood, although relaxation of the smooth muscle of the stomach probably plays a role. The rapid rise of human chorionic gonadotropin (hCG) also has been implicated, because the highest prevalence of nausea and vomiting occurs at a time in pregnancy when hCG levels are at their peak. Although in the past various theories have been put forth invoking a psychological cause of hyperemesis gravidarum, evidence for such an etiology is unconvincing (Buckwalter 2002). Hyperemesis gravidarum is the most extreme manifestation of nausea and vomiting. It usually is diagnosed when there is persistent nausea and vomiting accompanied by significant weight loss and ketonuria. Liver function tests and electrolytes may also be abnormal (American College of Obstetricians and Gynecologists 2004). Hyperemesis gravidarum is associated with molar pregnancy, which often manifests with hCG levels in the hundreds of thousands. The association between female sex of the fetus and hyperemesis gravidarum is not understood but is a known fact. In a retrospective study based on case notes of 166 women hospitalized for hyperemesis (Tan 2006), female fetuses were significantly associated with severe starvation ketonemia and high urea. When vomiting resulted in severe dehydration during pregnancy, 85% of the fetuses were female. In a study assessing the utility of acupuncture (Heazell 2006) to eliminate the symptoms of hyperemesis, no significant effect was observed compared with the use of antiemetic medication. Infants of mothers who do not have diabetes, with hyperemesis gravidarum, tend to have lower birth weight and may be small for gestational age (Bailit 2005, Dodds 2006), while such a relationship does not appear to be present for less severe nausea and vomiting. Special attention should be paid in a diabetic woman with hyperemesis gravidarum to ensure strict glucose control and hydration to prevent first-trimester complications associated with diabetes.

Typically, the symptoms begin before 9 weeks of gestation. The degree of nausea or vomiting a patient experiences and the sights or smells that trigger it can vary greatly from one pregnancy to another, although women who have had the problem before are more likely to experience it again. If it is a multiple gestation, symptoms are often more severe. When nausea and vomiting are first manifest after the first trimester or persist for >2–3 months, potential underlying causes should be given serious consideration; in women with diabetes gastroparesis should be high on the differential diagnosis list. Hyperthyroidism, gastrointestinal disorders, and genitourinary disorders also may cause hyperemesis.

## NONPHARMACOLOGIC TREATMENT

The treatment of morning sickness is seldom so successful that a woman will have complete relief. Time seems to be the only real cure. Women taking multivitamins at the time of conception are less likely to experience nausea and vomiting (Czeizel 1992, Emelianova 1999). Dietary changes may minimize the discomfort and make the situation at least manageable (Table 5.1), although evidence is lacking for most of these interventions. In a systematic review of published studies, ginger capsules (250–1500 mg per day) have been shown to improve nausea and vomiting (Borrelli 2005).

### Table 5.1 Tips for Controlling Nausea

- Remain hydrated:
  - Sip fluids throughout the day (water, decaffeinated tea, ice chips)
  - Maintain electrolytes, choosing lemonade, broth, diluted juice, ginger ale, popsicles, fruit ices
- Avoid an empty stomach:
  - Eat small frequent meals or snacks every 1–2 h.
  - Include protein snacks (e.g., hard-cooked eggs, nuts)
  - Keep simple, dry carbohydrate foods bedside (e.g., Cheerios, saltines)
  - Combine nutrients when possible, such as carbohydrate with protein (e.g., yogurt)
  - Eating salty and sweet combinations is sometimes effective (e.g., lemonade and pretzels)
  - Include a bedtime snack to reduce risk of early morning nausea
- Avoid an overly full stomach:
  - Separate intake of fluids and solid food
  - Avoid large meals
  - Avoid fatty foods
  - Avoid foods with strong odors and flavors
  - Take a prenatal vitamin at dinner or bedtime
  - Temporarily discontinue prenatal vitamins and use a children's chewable tablet and a folic acid supplement
  - Anemic women should continue iron, perhaps in divided doses
- Avoid caffeine

Nausea usually is worse when the stomach is empty—hence the early morning symptoms. For this reason, it is suggested that patients keep some starch, such as melba toast, rice cakes, saltines, or other low-fat crackers, at the bedside so they can eat if they become nauseated in the middle of the night or before getting out of bed in the morning. Eating a protein and carbohydrate snack at bedtime, such as cheese and crackers or half of a sandwich, will help prevent early morning nausea. This snack also helps prevent the development of ketonuria, which may aggravate nausea. To keep the stomach full, recommend to your patients that they eat six small meals per day. Generally, each meal should include food sources of carbohydrate, protein, and fat.

Women should consume what appeals to them and avoid foods that cause aversion. Tolerance of specific foods with nausea and vomiting of pregnancy is highly individual. Keeping stable blood glucose levels is an additional concern. Matching rapid-acting insulin to carbohydrates consumed is useful. Some women with diabetes are able to stabilize blood glucose and intake with the use of liquid nutritional supplements, if tolerated. Other lifestyle factors, such as adequate rest and social support, may affect symptoms of nausea and vomiting. Some women may have preexisting gastroparesis and require additional individualization of the meal plan.

Caffeine also may aggravate nausea, so advise a reduction in caffeine consumption. Fried, spicy, and fatty foods increase nausea. Peppers, chilies, and garlic are often culprits. Eating certain foods, or even simply smelling their aroma, can precipitate nausea, so advise patients to avoid these foods until the morning sickness has subsided. It may help if meals can be prepared by someone else. Taking prenatal vitamins after dinner or before bed may help decrease morning sickness.

## INSULIN ADJUSTMENTS

Women with gestational diabetes who are treated with diet alone usually can manage their morning sickness with dietary remedies. The management of women with type 1 diabetes (T1D) or insulin-treated type 2 diabetes (T2D) who experience morning sickness provides a challenge for even the most skilled practitioners.

Nausea may be a symptom of hypoglycemia, and hypoglycemia often aggravates nausea. It is therefore essential to have your patients check their blood glucose often to avoid hypoglycemia.

It is important that patients carry food at all times so that they can promptly treat any hypoglycemia or nausea. If nausea becomes severe enough to cause vomiting, women receiving insulin may need adjustments in the interval between their injection and meal.

The following approaches can be taken for decreasing premeal hypoglycemia and nausea:

- Recommend that patients take rapid-acting insulin after eating, once blood glucose levels begin to rise.
- Have patients take a portion of the insulin with a small part of the meal's carbohydrate to see how well the food is tolerated before taking the remainder of the insulin and the meal.

If a patient cannot tolerate food and has vomited after a meal, recommend that she initially substitute tomato juice for the meal (12 oz juice has 15 g carbohydrate), because fluids may be tolerated more easily. Once the vomiting has subsided, she can eat the remainder of the meal. Advise patients who have vomited to check their blood glucose and urine ketone levels frequently.

## MEDICAL MANAGEMENT

If vomiting during pregnancy is not controlled by dietary remedies and becomes severe, various medications often are prescribed (Niebyl 2010). Pyridoxine (vitamin B6), 10–25 mg orally every 8 h, was more effective than placebo in randomized trials (Sahakian 1991, Vutyavanich 1995) and is available over the counter. A combination of pyridoxine and an antihistamine, doxylamine, was popular and apparently effective, but was taken off the market in the U.S. because of lawsuits alleging teratogenicity, a concern not supported by data. It is still marketed in Canada, and caregivers in the U.S. may prescribe the two components separately, adding doxylamine 12.5–25 mg every 8 h if pyridoxine alone is unsuccessful. Doxylamine is available over the counter as Unisom Sleep Tabs, which contain 25 mg. Other antihistamines, such as diphenhydramine, meclizine, or dimenhydrinate, also may be prescribed. All of the antihistamines may cause drowsiness. When these approaches are not effective, prochlorperazine or promethazine may be used orally or rectally. Ondansetron 4–8 mg orally every 6 h is quite effective and the availability of a generic version has rendered this drug less costly than in the past. Metoclopramide 10 mg every 6 h may be effective (Matok 2009, Tan 2010), and is particularly helpful in women with diabetic gastroparesis, many of whom will experience persistent nausea and vomiting well beyond the first trimester. Many practitioners advise hospitalization to prevent dehydration, electrolyte disturbances, and weight loss. It is best to recommend hospitalization if vomiting continues for 8 h, the patient has persistent hypoglycemia, or the patient has developed significant ketonuria. Treatment usually consists of intravenous fluids, potassium replacement, and close monitoring of blood glucose, urine ketones, and weight. Antiemetic medications also may be needed until the cycle of vomiting has been stopped.

Persistent nausea and vomiting during pregnancy that is severe enough to cause large ketonuria and weight loss of ~5% is known as hyperemesis gravidarum. Hyperemesis occurs in 0.5–2.0% of pregnant women (American College of Obstetricians and Gynecologists 2004). Laboratory evaluation of such patients may include liver and pancreatic enzymes (which may be elevated), and electrolytres (which may reveal metabolic alkalosis). Intravenous rehydration is generally necessary, and hospitalization may be required, particularly in women with diabetes. Once stabilization has occurred, the patient may be maintained as an outpatient even if enteral tube feeding or parenteral nutrition is necessary to maintain body weight in severe cases. The mother's blood glucose levels should be kept in the normal range despite the intravenous therapy.

The best reassurance for patients is that the "tincture of time" is the best medicine. For most women, symptoms generally are lessened once they have eaten and are diminished markedly by the end of the fourth month. Women experiencing morning sickness are statistically less likely to experience a spontaneous loss or preterm birth (Weigel 1989). This can be especially reassuring information for women with diabetes.

## SELECTED READING

American College of Obstetricians and Gynecologists: Nausea and vomiting of pregnancy. ACOG Practice Bulletin No. 52. *Obstet Gynecol* 103:803–815, 2004 (reaffirmed 2011)

## REFERENCES

American College of Obstetricians and Gynecologists: Nausea and vomiting of pregnancy. ACOG Practice Bulletin No. 52. *Obstet Gynecol* 103:803–815, 2004 (reaffirmed 2011)

Bailit JL: Hyperemesis gravidarium: epidemiologic findings from a large cohort. *Am J Obstet Gynecol* 193:811–884, 2005

Borrelli F, Capasso R, Aviello G, Pittler MH, Izzo AA: Effectiveness and safety of ginger in the treatment of pregnancy-induced nausea and vomiting. *Obstet Gynecol* 105:849–856, 2005

Buckwalter JG, Simpson SW: Psychological factors in the etiology and treatment of severe nausea and vomiting in pregnancy. *Am J Obstet Gynecol* 186:s210–s214, 2002

Czeizel AE, Dudas I, Fritz G, Tecsoi A, Hanck A, Kunovitz G: The effect of periconceptional multivitamin-mineral supplementation on vertigo, nausea and vomiting in the first trimester of pregnancy. *Arch Gynecol Obstet* 251:181–185, 1992

Dodds L, Fell DB, Joseph KS, Allen VM, Butler B: Outcomes of pregnancies complicated by hyperemesis gravidarum. *Obstet Gynecol* 107:285–292, 2006

Emelianova S, Mazzotta P, Einarson A, Koren G: Prevalence and severity of nausea and vomiting of pregnancy and effect of vitamin supplementation. *Clin Invest Med* 22:106–110, 1999

Heazell A, Thorneycroft J, Walton V, Etherington I: Acupressure for the inpatient treatment of nausea and vomiting in early pregnancy: a randomized control trial. *Am J Obstet Gynecol* 194:815–820, 2006

Matok I, Gorodischer R, Koren G, Sheiner E, Wiznitzer A, Levy A: The safety of metoclopramide use in the first trimester of pregnancy. *N Engl J Med* 360:2528–2535, 2009

Niebyl JR: Nausea and vomiting in pregnancy. *N Engl J Med* 363:1544–1550, 2010

Sahakian V, Rouse D, Sipes S, Rose N, Niebyl J: Vitamin B6 is effective therapy for nausea and vomiting of pregnancy: a randomized, double-blind placebo-controlled study. *Obstet Gynecol* 78:33–36, 1991

Tan PC, Jacob R, Quek KF, Omar SZ: The fetal sex ratio and metabolic, bio-chemical, haematological and clinical indicators of severity of hyperemesis gravidarum. *Br J Obstet Gynaecol* 113:733–737, 2006

Tan PC, Khine PP, Vallikkannu N, Omar SZ: Promethazine compared with meto-clopramide for hyperemesis gravidarum: a randomized controlled trial. *Obstet Gynecol* 115:975–981, 2010

Vutyavanich T, Wongtra-ngan S, Ruangsri R: Pyridoxine for nausea and vomiting of pregnancy: a randomized, double-blind, placebo-controlled trial. *Am J Obstet Gynecol* 173:881–884, 1995

Weigel MM, Weigel RM: Nausea and vomiting of early pregnancy and preg-nancy outcome: an epidemiological study. *Br J Obstet Gynaecol* 96:1304–1311, 1989

# Nutrition Management of Preexisting Diabetes During Pregnancy

Highlights

Medical Nutrition Therapy

Weight Gain Recommendations

Macronutrients
Energy
Carbohydrate
Dietary Fiber
Glycemic Index
Resistant Starch and High-Amylose Foods
Protein
Dietary Fat

Micronutrients
Sodium
Folate
Iron
Vitamin D and Calcium
Other Nutrients

Meal Planning
Vitamin and Mineral Supplementation

Other Substances
Caffeine
Alcohol
Nonnutritive Sweeteners
Herbal Medicines and Supplements

# Highlights
# Nutrition Management of Preexisting Diabetes During Pregnancy

■ Most successful models of care include a multidisciplinary team with the woman with diabetes at the center.

■ Medical nutrition therapy should be provided by a registered dietitian and should include an individualized meal plan.

■ Weight gain recommendations are individualized, based on the Institute of Medicine revised BMI categories.

■ Nutrient needs of pregnant women with diabetes are based on the Institute of Medicine's 2006 Dietary Reference Intakes for Women, summarized in Table 6.2.

■ An overview of nutrition management of postpartum and lactating women with preexisting diabetes is included.

# Nutrition Management of Preexisting Diabetes During Pregnancy

Adequate nutrition is one of the most important influences on the health of pregnant women and their infants. Maintaining a good nutritional status optimizes maternal health and reduces the risk of birth defects and suboptimal fetal growth and lowers the risk of chronic health problems in their children (American Dietetic Association 2008). In pregnant women with preexisting diabetes (PDM), excellent glucose control from the first trimester and continued throughout pregnancy is associated with the lowest frequency of maternal fetal and neonatal complications (Kitzmiller 2008). Optimal glucose control, both before and early in pregnancy complicated by diabetes, has been shown to improve perinatal outcomes (Jovanovic 2005). Population surveys looking at infants of women with type 1 diabetes (T1D) indicated an excessive rate of macrosomia (birth weight >4,000 or >4,500 g) compared with the general population (Johnstone 2006).

The profound effects of changes in maternal metabolism during pregnancy on women with diabetes necessitate intensive management. The most successful models of care include a multidisciplinary team with the woman with diabetes as the center (American Diabetes Association 2008a, Kitzmiller 2008). Individualized medical nutrition therapy (MNT) should be provided, preferably, by a registered dietitian with knowledge of MNT specifically for pregnancy and diabetes (Reader 2006; American Diabetes Association 2004, 2008a, 2008b, 2010; Kitzmiller 2008). All members of the clinical team should understand and support the individualized meal plan. The pregnant woman should be a primary active member of the treatment team. The diabetes management team may guide, educate, and support the pregnant woman with diabetes, but she must manage her diet, perform self-monitoring of blood glucose (SMBG) levels, and keep extensive records. Pregnant women often are excited and motivated to make healthy lifestyle changes for their developing baby. Pregnancy visits can provide an opportunity to educate the woman with diabetes to adjust her diet to reduce the risk of, or to better manage, concurrent complications of PDM and improve long-term health.

## MEDICAL NUTRITION THERAPY

The goals of MNT for pregnancy in women with diabetes are to provide adequate nutrients for maternal and fetal needs while minimizing pregnancy complications, to promote appropriate weight gain, and to maintain optimal glucose control (Kitzmiller 2008). The current nutrient requirements for pregnant women with diabetes are similar to those for the nondiabetic pregnant population and are based on the Dietary Reference Intakes (DRIs), which are summarized in the Institute of Medicine's (IOM) *Dietary Reference Intakes: The Essential Guide to Nutrient Requirements* (Institute of Medicine, Food and Nutrition Board 2006). DRIs for nonpregnant, pregnant, and lactating women are found in Table 6.1. Weight gain recommendations for pregnancy were reviewed by the IOM in 2009 for the first time since 1990. The guidelines are based on observational data showing that women who gained weight within the IOM (1990) recommendations had better pregnancy outcomes compared with those who gained weight above or below recommendations (National Research Council 2009). This updated consensus report, *Weight Gain during Pregnancy: Reexamining the Guidelines*, acknowledges the need for individualized weight gain goals and has developed recommendations for obese women. As noted in the extensive review of these topics in *Management of Preexisiting Diabetes and Pregnancy* (Kitzmiller 2008), more research is needed to determine whether women with PDM have specific nutrient needs and weight gain recommendations that differ from the general pregnant population.

## WEIGHT GAIN RECOMMENDATIONS

Gaining the appropriate amount of weight during pregnancy enhances maternal and fetal well-being, while avoiding excessive postpartum weight retention, which can have implications for the long-term health of women and their children. Women who are becoming pregnant today do so at higher body weights than in the past. Studies continue to demonstrate that a woman's pregravid weight and gestational weight gain affects perinatal outcomes (Kitzmiller 2008, Dennedy 2012). The IOM (2009) recommendations (Table 6.2) evaluate weight gain during pregnancy from the perspective that factors affecting pregnancy begin before conception and continue through the first year after delivery. The weight gain guidelines are based on revised BMI categories and now have a specific recommendation for obese women. To meet the recommendations of the guidelines, women need to gain within the weight gain ranges for their BMI category.

Timing and rate of weight gain also affect outcomes. In the first trimester, relatively small amounts of weight gain are required (1.1–4.4 lb) (National Research Council 2009). In nondiabetic women, weight gain in the first half of pregnancy is a determinant of fetal linear growth. In the second and third trimesters, inadequate weight gain in normal weight and underweight nondiabetic women may be associated with premature birth or small-for-gestational-age (SGA) babies. In overweight and obese women, excessive weight gain is associated with an increased rate of fetal macrosomia, birth trauma, and increased cesarean section rate (Kitzmiller 2008). In women with diabetes, excessive weight gain can promote fetal overgrowth and fat deposition and has been associated with an increase in cesarean deliveries. It has been suggested that women with diabetes target weight gain totals at the lower end of the IOM's recommended weight gain range for BMI category. Weight loss is not recommended, but women with PDM who are obese and consuming adequate calories and nutrients (as evidenced by review of detailed food records) may not need to reach minimum weight gain recommendations (Institute of Medicine Food and Nutrition Board 1990). More research is needed in pregnant women with PDM to determine the effects of pregravid BMI, gestational weight gain, and weight retention on perinatal outcomes.

## Table 6.1 Dietary Reference Intakes for Women[a,b]

| Nutrient | Adult woman | Pregnancy | Lactation (0–6 months) |
|---|---|---|---|
| Energy (kcal) | 2,403 | 2,743[c], 2,855[d] | 2,698 |
| Protein (g/kg/d) | 0.8 | 1.1 | 1.1 |
| Carbohydrate (g/d) | 130 | 175 | 210 |
| Total fiber (g/d) | 25 | 28 | 29 |
| Fluids, l/day (cups/d) | 2.2 (~9) | 2.3 (~10) | 3.1 (~13) |
| Linoleic acid (g/d) | 12 | 13 | 13 |
| α-Linolenic acid (g/d) | 12 | 13 | 13 |
| Vitamin A (µg RAE)[e] | 700 | 770 | 1,300 |
| Vitamin D (µg)[f,g] | 10 | 10 | 10 |
| Vitamin E (mg α-tocopherol) | 15 | 15 | 19 |
| Vitamin K (µg) | 90 | 90 | 90 |
| Vitamin C (mg) | 75 | 85 | 120 |
| Thiamin (mg) | 1.1 | 1.4 | 1.4 |
| Riboflavin (mg) | 1.1 | 1.4 | 1.6 |
| Vitamin B-6 (mg) | 1.3 | 1.9 | 2.0 |
| Niacin (mg NE)[h] | 14 | 18 | 17 |
| Folate (µg dietary folate equivalents) | 400 | 600 | 500 |
| Vitamin B12 (µg) | 2.4 | 2.6 | 2.8 |
| Pantothenic acid (mg) | 5 | 6 | 7 |
| Biotin (µg) | 30 | 30 | 35 |
| Choline (mg) | 425 | 450 | 550 |
| Calcium (mg) | 1,000 | 1,000 | 1,000 |
| Phosphorus (mg) | 700 | 700 | 700 |
| Magnesium (mg) | 320 | 350 | 310 |
| Iron (mg) | 18 | 27 | 19 |
| Zinc (mg) | 8 | 11 | 12 |
| Iodine (µg) | 150 | 220 | 290 |
| Selenium (µg) | 55 | 60 | 70 |
| Fluoride (mg) | 3 | 3 | 3 |
| Manganese (mg) | 1.8 | 2.0 | 2.6 |
| Molybdenum (µg) | 45 | 50 | 50 |
| Chromium (µg) | 25 | 30 | 45 |

*(continues p. 82)*

## Table 6.1 Dietary Reference Intakes for Women[a,b] *(continued)*

| Nutrient | Adult woman | Pregnancy | Lactation (0–6 months) |
|---|---|---|---|
| Copper (µg) | 900 | 1,000 | 1,300 |
| Sodium (mg) | 2,300 | 2,300 | 2,300 |
| Potassium (mg) | 4,700 | 4,700 | 5,100 |

[a] Data from Institute of Medicine Food and Nutrition Board: *Dietary Reference Intakes: The Essential Guide to Nutrient Requirements*. Washington, DC, The National Academies Press, 2006; Institute of Medicine Food and Nutrition Board: *Dietary Reference Intakes for Calcium and Vitamin D*. Washington, DC, National Academy Press, 2010

[b] Values are recommended dietary allowances except energy (estimated energy requirement) and total fiber, linoleic acid, α-linolenic acid, vitamin K, pantothenic acid, biotin, choline, manganese, chromium, sodium, and potassium (adequate intakes).

[c] Second trimester for women ages 19–50 years.

[d] Third trimester for women ages 19–50 years.

[e] RAE = retinol activity equivalents.

[f] As cholecalciferol: 1 µg cholecalciferol = 40 IU vitamin D.

[g] Under the assumption of minimal sunlight.

[h] NE = niacin equivalents: 1 mg niacin = 60 mg tryptophan.

Many BMI calculators are available; one such site is cdc.gov/healthyweight/assessingbmi/adult_bmi/english_bmi_calculator/bmi_calculator.html.

Height and weight should be measured at the first prenatal visit (American College of Obstetricians and Gynecologists 2005). Care should be taken to assess height accurately, but pregravid weight status is often subjective information. An accurate height–weight history may be available from health records and can be supportive data. If the woman with diabetes has had preconception counseling, this information may be more readily available. When reported pregravid weight is not reasonable based on current weight and gestational age, an estimated weight can be utilized. BMI category can then be assigned. Weight should be monitored at each visit (American College of Obstetricians and Gynecologists 2005, American Diabetes Association 2008a). Patterns of gain can be plotted using prenatal weight gain grids based on the IOM's recommended ranges. This tool can be used to educate and motivate the pregnant women with diabetes to engage in efforts to gain the appropriate amounts of weight (see Selected Readings). Women who have gained excessive amounts of weight early in gestation should not be severely restricted, but weight gain may be slowed and weight loss should be encouraged for the postpartum period (Kitzmiller 2008).

## MACRONUTRIENTS

Adequate intake of energy from carbohydrate, fiber, protein, and fat are necessary to support fetal-placental growth and provide for maternal needs and fat storage. These nutrients also have a strong impact on glucose control and pregnancy success for women with diabetes.

The IOM's DRIs are the recommended guidelines for nutrient intake for all stages of the life cycle, including pregnancy (Institute of Medicine Food and Nutrition Board 2006). Values are provided for individual macro- and micronutrients in Table 6.1. It is noted that women eat foods, not nutrients in isolation. Incorporating a woman's food preferences and tolerances, while encouraging consumption of a wholesome, balanced meal plan is a key component of MNT for pregnant women with diabetes.

## Table 6.2 IOM Recommendations for Rate of Weight Gain

| Prepregnancy BMI (kg/m²) | Total weight gain (lb) | Rates of weight gain second and third trimester (lb/week) |
|---|---|---|
| Underweight (<18.5) | 28–40 | 1 (1–1.3) |
| Normal weight (18.5–24.9) | 25–35 | 1 (0.8–1) |
| Overweight (25.0–29.9) | 15–25 | 0.6 (0.5–0.7) |
| Obese (≥30.0) | 11–20 | 0.5 (0.4–0.6) |

Adapted from National Research Council: *Weight Gain During Pregnancy: Reexamining the Guidelines*. Washington, DC, The National Academies Press, 2009

## ENERGY

Most pregnant women need between 2,200 kcal and 2,900 kcal a day to meet their nutritional needs (American Dietetic Association 2008). This should be adjusted taking into consideration prepregnancy BMI, rate of weight gain, maternal age, and appetite (Tables 6.3 and 6.4). Energy requirements for pregnancy are based on the estimated energy requirements (EER) of nonpregnant women with adjustments for pregnancy (Institute of Medicine Food and Nutrition Board 2006).

## Table 6.3 Estimated Energy Requirement (kcal/day) Formula

| Physical activity | PA value | Activity examples |
|---|---|---|
| Sedentary | 1.0 | Daily living activities (e.g., household tasks, walking to the bus) |
| Low active | 1.12 | Daily living activities + 30–60 min daily moderate activity (e.g., walking at 5–7 km/h) |
| Active | 1.27 | Daily living activities + at least 60 min daily moderate activity |
| Very active | 1.45 | Daily living activities + 60 min daily moderate activity + an additional 60 min of strenuous activity, or 120 min of moderate activity |

Nonpregnant Woman (19–50 years old)

EER = [354 − (6.91 x age [years]) + PA* x [(9.36 x weight [kg]) + (726 x height [m])]

* Physical Activity (PA) Coefficients

Adapted from Institute of Medicine Food and Nutrition Board: *Dietary Reference Intakes: The Essential Guide to Nutrient Requirements*. Washington, DC, The National Academies Press, 2006

## Table 6.4 Energy Adjustments for Pregnancy

| | |
|---|---|
| First Trimester | EER + 0 kcal/day |
| Second Trimester | EER + 340 kcal/day |
| Third Trimester | EER + 452 kcal/day |
| Third Trimester | EER + 452 kcal/day |

EER = estimated energy requirements.
Adapted from Institute of Medicine Food and Nutrition Board: *Dietary Reference Intakes: The Essential Guide to Nutrient Requirements*. Washington, DC, The National Academies Press, 2006

Energy needs may be highly variable and an individualized approach is recommended (American Diabetes Association 2008a, Kitzmiller 2008). With the prevalence of obesity and the importance of controlled weight gain, some women with PDM may benefit from a reduced energy intake. Studies based on women with gestational diabetes mellitus (GDM) have reported good outcomes with energy intakes of 1,700–1,800 kcal/day (limitation of 30%) (Dornhurst 1991). Moderately limiting energy also may be beneficial for women with type 2 diabetes (T2D) who are obese and with insulin resistance. More severe restrictions of 1,200–1,600 kcal may lead to weight loss or starvation ketosis, which should be avoided (Knopp 1991). Close monitoring of interval weight gains can allow for the adjustment of the energy level of the meal plan. If weight gains are below or above the target range, a discussion can be initiated with the women regarding an action plan to adjust energy intake and physical activity.

### CARBOHYDRATE

Glucose is the preferred fuel for fetal growth and development. Carbohydrate is the primary nutrient affecting maternal glucose levels. The recommended daily allowance (RDA) for an adult woman is 130 g/day of digestible carbohydrate based on the minimum amounts of glucose utilized by the brain. Minimum carbohydrate recommendations for pregnant women increase to 175 g/day to meet fetal needs (Institute of Medicine Food and Nutrition Board 2006). Carbohydrates (sugars, starches, and fiber) are found in fruits, vegetables, whole grains, legumes, milk, and yogurt and the added sugars in the foods we consume. The Food and Nutrition Board has set the acceptable macronutrient distribution range (AMDR) for carbohydrate for all populations, including pregnant women, at 45–65% of total calories. In women with diabetes, carbohydrate frequently is limited to 40–60% of total calories to meet postprandial blood glucose goals, but it should include the minimum recommendation of 175 g/day of digestible carbohydrate (Kitzmiller 2008). It may be difficult to meet the other nutritional needs of pregnancy when carbohydrate is limited to the minimum requirement. The amount of carbohydrate should be individualized based on patient preferences; weight gain goals; insulin doses; and premeal, postmeal, and nighttime glucose values.

The type of carbohydrate consumed also affects postprandial blood glucose levels. Extrinsic variables may influence postprandial blood glucose values, including fasting or preprandial blood glucose levels, macronutrient distribution of foods consumed, available insulin, and insulin resistance. To meet the nutrient needs of pregnancy, meals and snacks are usually a combination of macronutrients, not only carbohydrate. Use of sucrose in a diabetes meal plan is acceptable (American Diabetes Association 2008b); in pregnancy, however, this should be limited because of the importance of a nutrient-dense diet and weight management. Use of sugar alcohols is permissible and only half of the total grams of carbohydrate should be calculated into the total carbohydrate load (Knopp 1991).

## Table 6.5 Selected Food Sources Ranked by Amount of Dietary Fiber and Calories per Standard Food Portion

| Food | Standard portion size | Calories in standard portion | Dietary fiber in standard portion (g) |
|---|---|---|---|
| Beans (navy, pinto, black, kidney, white, great northern, lima), cooked | 1/2 cup | 104–149 | 6.2–9.6 |
| Bran, ready-to-eat cereal (100%) | 1/3 cup (about 1 ounce) | 81 | 9.1 |
| Split peas, lentils, chickpeas, or cowpeas, cooked | 1/2 cup | 108–134 | 5.6–8.1 |
| Artichoke, cooked | 1/2 cup hearts | 45 | 7.2 |
| Pear | 1 medium | 103 | 5.5 |
| Soybeans, mature, cooked | 1/2 cup | 149 | 5.2 |
| Plain rye wafer crackers | 2 wafers | 73 | 5.0 |
| Bran, ready-to-eat cereals (various) | 1/3–3/4 cup (about 1 ounce) | 88–91 | 2.6–5.0 |
| Asian pear | 1 small | 51 | 4.4 |
| Green peas, cooked | 1/2 cup | 59–67 | 3.5–4.4 |
| Whole-wheat English muffin | 1 muffin | 134 | 4.4 |
| Bulgur, cooked | 1/2 cup | 76 | 4.1 |
| Mixed vegetables, cooked | 1/2 cup | 59 | 4.0 |
| Raspberries | 1/2 cup | 32 | 4.0 |
| Sweet potato, baked in skin | 1 medium | 103 | 3.8 |
| Blackberries | 1/2 cup | 31 | 3.8 |
| Soybeans, green, cooked | 1/2 cup | 127 | 3.8 |
| Prunes, stewed | 1/2 cup | 133 | 3.8 |
| Shredded wheat, ready-to-eat cereal | 1/2 cup (about 1 ounce) | 95–100 | 2.7–3.8 |
| Figs, dried | 1/4 cup | 93 | 3.7 |

| Food | Standard portion size | Calories in standard portion | Dietary fiber in standard portion (g) |
|---|---|---|---|
| Apple, with skin | 1 small | 77 | 3.6 |
| Pumpkin, canned | 1/2 cup | 42 | 3.6 |
| Greens (spinach, collards, turnip greens), cooked | 1/2 cup | 14–32 | 2.5–3.5 |
| Almonds | 1 ounce | 163 | 3.5 |
| Sauerkraut, canned | 1/2 cup | 22 | 3.4 |
| Whole wheat spaghetti, cooked | 1/2 cup | 87 | 3.1 |
| Banana | 1 medium | 105 | 3.1 |
| Orange | 1 medium | 62 | 3.1 |
| Guava | 1 fruit | 37 | 3.0 |
| Potato, baked, with skin | 1 small | 128 | 3.0 |
| Oat bran muffin | 1 small | 178 | 3.0 |
| Pearled barley, cooked | 1/2 cup | 97 | 3.0 |
| Dates | 1/4 cup | 104 | 2.9 |
| Winter squash, cooked | 1/2 cup | 38 | 2.9 |
| Parsnips, cooked | 1/2 cup | 55 | 2.8 |
| Tomato paste | 1/4 cup | 54 | 2.7 |
| Broccoli, cooked | 1/2 cup | 26–27 | 2.6–2.8 |
| Okra, cooked from frozen | 1/2 cup | 26 | 2.6 |

From U.S. Department of Agriculture, Center for Nutrition Policy and Promotion: *Report of the Dietary Guidelines Advisory Committee on the Dietary Guidelines for Americans,* 2010. Available at http://www.fda.gov/dietary-guidelines.

## DIETARY FIBER

Recommendations for adequate intake (AI) of dietary fiber during pregnancy are 28 g/day of digestible fiber (Institute of Medicine Food and Nutrition Board 2006) (Table 6.5). Increasing dietary fiber intake in people with diabetes who are not pregnant has a beneficial effect on lipids (American Diabetes Association 2008b). In some studies of pregnant women with T1D and GDM, there is evidence that the second- and third-trimester insulin dosage was correlated negatively with dietary fiber intake, but others found no association (Kitzmiller 2008). Adequate fiber intake can minimize the risk of, or alleviate, the common pregnancy complaint of constipation, which is the result of slowed digestion. Inclusion of adequate fiber also may increase satiety and aid in the management of appetite.

Many pregnant women, including those with diabetes, consume less than recommended amounts of fiber. When counseling pregnant women to increase fiber, the changes should be made incrementally. A dramatic increase may trigger gastrointestinal discomfort and discourage women from making healthy changes. Pregnant women with diabetes do not need more fiber than women who do not have diabetes, but they should be encouraged to include fiber-rich foods to meet the recommendation. If a food has >5 g dietary fiber, subtract half that amount from the total carbohydrates for insulin bolusing (Wheeler 2008).

## GLYCEMIC INDEX

The glycemic index (GI) is a ranking of foods based on a specific carbohydrate amount and the postprandial incremental glucose response and insulin demand. This measures quality, but not quantity. The concept of glycemic load compares the overall effect of a usual portion of food. In practice, the postprandial blood glucose level is measuring the glucose level of an entire meal. A small, randomized controlled study in women with GDM concluded that there were no differences in key pregnancy outcomes with consumption of a low-GI diet versus a conventional high-fiber diet (Louie 2011). Another small study in GDM demonstrated use of a low-GI diet may reduce the number of women requiring insulin therapy (Barker 2009). GI or glucose level can be used as an additional tool for individuals to use to improve glucose control based on postprandial results. A glucose level exchange list is available in *Management of Preexisiting Diabetes and Pregnancy* (Kitzmiller 2008) and may be useful. More studies are needed in pregnant women with PDM.

## RESISTANT STARCH AND HIGH-AMYLOSE FOODS

Naturally occurring nondigestible oligosaccharides or foods produced by the modification of starch during processing are termed "resistant starches." There is some evidence that these foods may have a beneficial effect on glucose control, but no long-term studies have been conducted on people with diabetes (American Diabetes Association 2008b, Wheeler 2008). Food sources include legumes, seeds, whole grains, high-amylose corn, cooked and chilled potatoes, pasta, and rice. Many of these foods are nutrient dense and may be included as healthy carbohydrate choices in the meal plan.

## PROTEIN

Additional protein, providing indispensable amino acids, is required during pregnancy for the expansion of maternal plasma volume and amniotic fluid and to support the growth of placental, fetal, and maternal tissue. The RDA for protein in the nonpregnant woman is 0.8 g/kg/day. During the second and third trimester, the requirement increases to 1.1 g/kg/day or an increase of ~25 g/day (Institute of Medicine, Food and Nutrition Board 2006). Protein sources include animal sources (meat, poultry, fish, eggs, milk, cheese, yogurt) and plants, grains, nuts, seeds, and vegetables. Protein has a minimal effect on postprandial glucose excursion and may be useful to provide satiety and necessary calories. Creating a meal plan for a pregnant woman with diabetes who practices a vegan eating style requires skill. Women who have overt nephropathy should meet the 1.1g/kg RDA for protein, but they should not consume <60 g/day (American Diabetes Association 2008a). For example, an 80-kg (176-lb) woman with nephropathy should limit her protein intake to 88 g/day, but a women weighing only 46 kg (101 lb) should meet the minimum recommendation of 60 g/day.

## DIETARY FAT

Intake of dietary fat provides energy and essential fatty acids, while enhancing absorption of fat-soluble vitamins. There is no RDA for total dietary fat intake. Excess fat intake, however, contributes significantly to energy intake. Fats provide more calories per gram than any other calorie source (9 calories per gram) and excess intake may result in excessive weight gain. This may lead to increased insulin resistance and postpartum weight retention in women with diabetes. It is also important to consider the long-term cardiovascular impact of fat intake in pregnant women with diabetes. Meal plans for women with diabetes generally contain 25–40% of daily calories from fat.

Types of fat include saturated (SFA), transunsaturated, monounsaturated (MUFA), and polyunsaturated fatty acids (PUFA). In the interest of long-term maternal health SFA, found primarily in animal products, should be limited to 7–10% of total calories (Institute of Medicine Food and Nutrition Board 2006, American Diabetes Association 2008a). *Trans* fat, primarily synthetic, intake should be minimal (Institute of Medicine Food and Nutrition Board 2010). Women with diabetes who have preexisting dyslipidemia should continue to limit their cholesterol intake to <200 mg/day. The remaining 20–30% of daily calories should come from MUFA (e.g., olive oil, avocado, canola oil, almonds) and PUFA (e.g., soybean, corn, and safflower oil).

The adequate intake for essential fatty acids in pregnancy is 13 g/day of omega-6 (n-6) fatty acids and 1.4 g/day of omega-3 (n-3) fatty acids (Institute of Medicine Food and Nutrition Board 2006). The key omega-3 (n-3) fatty acids include eicosapentaenoic acid (EPA) and docosahexaenoic acid (DHA). DHA is a PUFA necessary for fetal central nervous system development. DHA is found mainly in cold-water fatty fish such as salmon. It is recommended that nonpregnant and pregnant women with diabetes eat at least two meals of oily ocean fish per week to reduce the risks of cardiovascular disease (CVD) and hypertriglyceridemia (American Diabetes Association 2008a, 2008b). In pregnancy, women should avoid eating fish potentially high in mercury and polychlorinated biphenyls (PCBs). By limiting consumption to 12 oz per week and avoiding consumption of large predatory fish (e.g., swordfish, king mackerel, shark, and tilefish) pregnant women can incorporate seafood in their diet (U.S. Department of Agriculture, Center for Nutrition Policy and Promotions 2012). Information regarding eating safe seafood can encourage women with diabetes to include healthy seafood choices for their long-term health and that of their developing fetus.

## MICRONUTRIENTS

## SODIUM

The sodium requirement during pregnancy is 2,300 mg daily, the same as for a nonpregnant adult woman without diabetes (Institute of Medicine Food and Nutrition Board 2006). The *Dietary Guidelines for Americans, 2010* (U.S. Department of Agriculture, Center for Nutrition Policy and Promotions 2012) state "virtually all Americans consume more sodium than they need," and recommend a reduction in salt intake in the U.S. population (Louie 2011). Pregnant women with diabetes may be encouraged to reduce sodium to recommended levels. According to the *Dietary Guidelines* (U.S. Department of Agriculture, Center for Nutrition Policy and Promotions 2012), some suggestions are as follows:

- Read the nutrition facts label for information on the sodium content of foods and purchase foods that are low in sodium.
- Consume more fresh foods and fewer processed foods that are high in sodium.
- Eat more home-prepared foods, where you have more control over sodium, and use little or no salt or salt-containing seasonings when cooking or eating foods.
- When eating at restaurants, ask that salt not be added to your food or order lower-sodium options.

## FOLATE

Folate functions as a coenzyme in the transfer of single carbon units from one compound to another. A folate deficiency during early gestation is associated with impaired cellular growth and replication resulting in fetal malformations, spontaneous abortions, preterm delivery, and low birth weight (Kitzmiller 2008). As a result of the evidence for the role of folate in the prevention of neural tube defects, the U.S. Public Health Service recommends that all women in the periconceptional period consume 400 µg of folic acid daily from a combination of supplements, fortified foods, and a varied diet. During pregnancy, folate requirements increase to 600 µg/day (Institute of Medicine Food and Nutrition Board 2009). Sources of food folate include oranges and orange juice, beans and peas, and dark green leafy vegetables. Folic acid is added to fortified foods, such as grain and cereal products.

Folate supplementation can mask vitamin $B_{12}$ deficiency in women with T1D who have autoimmune gastritis or malabsorption (American Diabetes Association 2008a). Obtaining baseline vitamin $B_{12}$ levels may be useful in these women. Vegetarian women also may need supplementation of vitamin $B_{12}$.

## IRON

The RDA for iron is 27 mg/day throughout pregnancy (Institute of Medicine Food and Nutrition Board 2006). Although iron absorption increases during pregnancy, extra iron is required for fetal erythropoesis and an increase in maternal red cell mass. Maternal iron deficiency anemia increases the risk of low birth weight, preterm delivery, and perinatal mortality (Institute of Medicine Food and Nutrition Board 2001). Iron supplementation should be initiated if there is laboratory evidence of anemia. In the first and third trimester, this is a hemoglobin of <11.0g/dl and in the second trimester it is a hemoglobin of <10.5 g/dl (American College of Obstetricians and Gynecologists 2008, American Diabetes Association 2008a). Women with anemia may need elemental iron supplementation of 60–120 mg/day for treatment.

## VITAMIN D AND CALCIUM

Vitamin D is necessary to maintain positive calcium homeostasis in pregnancy. A maternal deficiency in vitamin D may lead to low serum calcium in the infant and adversely affect neonatal bone metabolism. Vitamin D is found in egg yolks, fatty fish, and fortified milk. Ready-to-eat breakfast cereals as well as some brands of orange juice, yogurt, margarine, and other food products are now fortified with vitamin D. Current interest and concern surrounding Vitamin D prompted the IOM to issue the consensus report *Dietary Reference Intakes for Vitamin D and Calcium* in 2010 (Institute of Medicine Food and Nutrition Board 2010). Calcium was included in the report due to its interrelationship with vitamin D. The RDA for vitamin D in pregnancy was set at 600 IU.

Calcium absorption increases in pregnancy. As a result, the RDA for calcium in pregnancy is 1,000 mg/day, the same as for nonpregnant individuals. Adequate calcium intake protects maternal bone mass. Good sources of calcium are milk, yogurt, and cheese. When a pregnant woman with diabetes does not consume adequate calcium from dairy sources, supplementation of 600 mg/day is recommended (Institute of Medicine Food and Nutrition Board 1990).

## OTHER NUTRIENTS

Chromium, magnesium, potassium, selenium, and zinc play critical roles in fetal development. Deficiencies in these nutrients also may affect carbohydrate tolerance (Kitzmiller 2008). Currently, there is no evidence to support a recommendation to routinely supplement pregnant women with diabetes with antioxidants vitamin C and vitamin E beyond the recommendations of the IOM for all pregnant women. It is important to counsel pregnant women with diabetes to eat healthful, nutrient-dense diets to achieve the DRIs for adequacy (see Table 6.2). An extensive review of specific nutrients is available in *Management of Preexisiting Diabetes and Pregnancy* (Kitzmiller 2008).

## MEAL PLANNING

MNT for pregnant women with diabetes includes an individualized assessment and meal plan (Table 6.6). This plan should "promote consumption of a wholesome balanced diet consistent with ethnic, cultural, and financial considerations" (American Diabetes Association 2008a ). A women's physical activity, food intake, and insulin therapy work in concert. The meal plan should provide nutrient adequacy, appropriate calorie level, usual eating schedule, and appropriate amount of carbohydrate at all meals and snacks. In pregnancy, women can experience pregnancy complaints, food aversions, intolerances, ptyalism, or pica, all of which can affect nutrient intake and glucose control. The meal plan also is constructed to avoid hypo- and hyperglycemia. Because of fetal demands for glucose, the pregnant woman with diabetes requiring insulin therapy may become hypoglycemic if she delays meals, skips a snack or meal, eats too little, exercises more than usual, or takes too much insulin.

## Table 6.6 Basic Meal Plan for Pregnancy and Lactation

| Food group | Minimum number of daily servings |
| --- | --- |
| Whole-grain breads, rice, pasta, cereal | 6–9 servings |
| Vegetables (include green leafy and yellow) | 4 servings |
| Fruits (include vitamin C source daily) | 3 servings |
| Milk, cheese, yogurt (low-fat) | 3 servings |
| Meat, fish, poultry (lean), dry beans, egg, and nuts | 2 servings |
| Oils (includes fat from nuts) | 6 tsp |

Adapted from U.S. Department of Agriculture, Center for Nutrition Policy and Promotion: *Report of the Dietary Guidelines Advisory Committee on the Dietary Guidelines for Americans, 2010.* Available at http://www.fns.usda.gov/dietary-guidelines.

The individualized meal plan for pregnant women with diabetes focuses on consistency. Macronutrients, including carbohydrate, are distributed evenly through the day, usually in three meals and two to four snacks. SMBG is an integral part of diabetes self-management. Keeping daily food and SMBG records provides invaluable information to guide treatment. Reviewing daily food records is ideal, but obtaining a series of days (three to five or more) before a visit can assist considerably in adjusting MNT and insulin doses. In the first trimester of diabetic pregnancy, especially with T1D, women may experience an increased incidence of hypoglycemia. Consistency in the meal plan can minimize this risk. Carbohydrate may be less well tolerated in the morning (American Diabetes Association 2008a), but results of SMBG can guide changes in either carbohydrate consumption or medication.

Women with diabetes can use a variety of methods to manage their carbohydrate intake. Some women "count" carbohydrate grams, some use portion sizes or "exchanges," some estimate portions based on experience or "my plate," and some use a combination of methods. The usual carbohydrate in a measured portion is 15 g. Daytime snacks usually are needed to prevent premeal low blood glucose levels and an adequate bedtime snack may reduce nocturnal hypoglycemia. Women on intensive management, after education, may use carbohydrate-to-insulin ratios to help manage blood glucose levels. The ratios need frequent adjustment as glucose tolerance varies with gestational age. According to the *Management of Preexisting Diabetes and Pregnancy* (Kitzmiller 2008), carbohydrate distribution for a typical meal plan for a pregnant woman with diabetes would include the following:

- Breakfast: 15–45 g carbohydrate
- Lunch: 30–75 g carbohydrate
- Dinner: 30–75 g carbohydrate
- Daytime snacks: 15–30 g carbohydrate
- Bedtime snack: 15–45 g carbohydrate

Close monitoring of food and SMBG records by the management team can help a woman meet her goals of excellent glycemia, adequate nutrients, and appropriate weight gain.

## VITAMIN AND MINERAL SUPPLEMENTATION

Multivitamin and mineral supplements are recommended for women with poor diets, with iron deficiency anemia, and who include little or no animal protein in their diets. Women with multiple pregnancies, with other high-risk conditions, and who use tobacco or abuse alcohol or drugs also should take a supplement. Pregnant women with diabetes may be supplemented to meet recommended levels of vitamins, minerals, and trace elements. Nutrient-dense food choices should be encouraged in all pregnant women with diabetes.

## OTHER SUBSTANCES

### CAFFEINE

High caffeine intake during pregnancy is associated with spontaneous miscarriage and low birth weight, but it has not been shown to correlate with birth defects. Reports have shown that large quantities of caffeine ingested (>300 mg/day) increase the risk of intrauterine growth restriction and spontaneous abortion (Higdon 2006). Pregnant women who consume caffeine-containing beverages should do so in moderation. The suggested limit is ≤300 mg caffeine daily (Table 6.7).

### ALCOHOL

Alcohol should not be consumed by pregnant women, including those with diabetes (Institute of Medicine Food and Nutrition Board 2006).

### NONNUTRITIVE SWEETENERS

Use of nonnutritive sweeteners classified as Generally Recognized as Safe are acceptable in moderation during pregnancy. These include acesulfame-K, aspartame, saccharin, stevia, sucralose, and neotame (American Dietetic Association 2008). Blends of artificial sweeteners that contain dextrose should be counted as carbohydrate in the meal plan.

## Table 6.7 Caffeine Content of Common Beverages

| Beverage | | Serving size | Caffeine (mg/serving) |
|---|---|---|---|
| Coffee, | brewed | 8 oz | 130 |
| | instant | 8 oz | 45 |
| | coffeehouse | 16 oz | 320 |
| Tea, | medium | 8 oz | 42 |
| | green | 8 oz | 30 |
| Energy drink | | 16 oz | 160 |
| Cola | | 12 oz | 35 |
| Energy shot | | 2 oz | 138 |

From EnergyFiend: Caffeine content of drinks and products. Available at http://www.energyfiend.com/the-caffeine-database. Accessed 10 August 2012; American Beverage Association: Caffeine comparison. Available at http://www.ameribev.org/nutrition--science/beverage-ingredients/caffeine. Accessed 10 August 2012

## HERBAL MEDICINES AND SUPPLEMENTS

Popular culture views herbal, "natural," botanical, or other supplements as safe. Different cultures may include use of these teas and other herbals routinely. Heath professionals should ask pregnant women with diabetes whether they use any of these substances so they may be evaluated for potential risk during pregnancy, including effects on blood glucose control (American Dietetic Association 2008).

## FOOD SAFETY

### LISTERIA

Women with diabetes are at risk for foodborne illness. Pregnant women are at high risk to become sick from listeria, a bacteria found in some foods. Infection can result in miscarriage, stillbirth, preterm delivery, or neonatal illness (U.S. Department of Agriculture, Food Safety 2011). To avoid infection pregnant women should not consume the following:

- Hot dogs, luncheon meats, or other deli meats unless they are reheated until steaming hot.
- Soft cheese such as Feta, queso blanco, queso fresco, Brie, Camembert, blue-veined cheeses, and Panela unless it is labeled as made with pasteurized milk.
- Salads made in the store such as ham salad, egg salad, chicken salad, tuna salad, or seafood salad.
- Raw or unpasteurized milk.
- Refrigerated paté, meat spreads, or smoked seafood (unless cooked). Shelf-stable or canned paté or meat spreads can be consumed.

## MERCURY

Women should follow the *Dietary Guidelines 2010* (U.S. Department of Agriculture, Center for Nutrition Policy and Promotion 2012) for inclusion of safe seafood as outlined above in the section Dietary Fat.

## POSTPARTUM NUTRITION MANAGEMENT

The nutritional quality of the diet of a woman with diabetes continues to remain important during the postpartum period. Women with T2D may return to pre-pregnancy oral antidiabetic medications or continue on insulin therapy. Women with T1D experience significant insulin dose reductions from the insulin doses required during the insulin-resistant state of pregnancy. Those with operative deliveries have additional nutritional demands for wound healing as well as the need for glucose control. Optimum blood glucose control may be encouraged by continuing SMBG and following the principles of the pregnancy meal plan.

During the postpartum period, the need for supplementation depends on the woman's nutritional status. Women found to be anemic after delivery or at their postpartum checkup should take 60–120 mg/day of elemental iron daily until the anemia is resolved. Some high-risk women may require a multivitamin–mineral supplement. Vegetarian women also may need supplementation of vitamin $B_{12}$ (Institute of Medicine Food and Nutrition Board 2006).

Women with diabetes who are overweight (BMI 25–30) or obese (BMI ≥30) should be encouraged to lose weight. Moderate weight loss and CVD risk reduction may be achieved by balancing caloric intake and physical activity (150 min/week) (American Diabetes Association 2012). Nutrition recommendations for managing diabetes in women may be implemented (American Diabetes Association 2008b). Women should be encouraged to continue healthy eating changes made during pregnancy to benefit lifelong health.

## LACTATION NUTRITION MANAGEMENT

Exclusive breast-feeding is recommended for the first 6 months of life and should continue, with supplemental calories, from 6–12 months of age (Reader 2004; American Academy of Pediatrics, Section on Breastfeeding 2005; American Dietetic Association 2009). The benefits of breast-feeding for women with diabetes and their infants are well established. Breast-feeding has been associated with a reduction of risk for development of diabetes in women with previous GDM and in the children of women with diabetes. A review of the current evidence on the associations of breast-feeding, formula feeding, and the early introduction of cow's milk and the development of T1D, suggests that short duration or lack of breast-feeding may be a risk factor for the development of T1D (Patelarou 2012). Early infant feeding patterns are being examined in the Trial to Reduce Type 1 Diabetes in the Genetically at Risk (TRIGR). TRIGR addresses short-term breast-feeding and early exposure to complex dietary proteins, such as cow's milk and cereal proteins, which have been implicated in β-cell autoimmunity, by weaning to a hydrolyzed formula in infancy (Knip 2011). The children in this study are being followed until age 10 years with the study to be unblinded in 2017. Children of women with diabetes (preexisting and GDM), who were breast-fed for ≥6 months had reduced adiposity compared with those who were not adequately breast-fed (Crume 2011). Short duration of breast-feeding (i.e., ≤4 months) and large birth weight are predictive factors for obesity in children of men and women with T1D (Hummel 2009). The benefits of breast-feeding are magnified by early initiation, duration, and exclusivity.

The majority of women with diabetes who are well controlled can successfully breast-feed. Predictive factors for the initiation and maintenance of breast-feeding in women with T1D include problems establishing early breast-feeding due to a higher degree of maternal and infant complications (Sparud-Lundin 2011). Women who are obese are less likely to breast-feed, and therefore frequent prenatal visits should be used as an opportunity to educate women and address potential barriers. Interventions to support successful breast-feeding in women with diabetes should be instituted. More research is needed on the specific benefits and challenges of breast-feeding for women with diabetes and their infants.

## NUTRITION RECOMMENDATIONS

The goals of MNT for lactation in women with diabetes are to provide excellent nutrition for the infant, promote maternal glucose control, and contribute to long-term risk reduction for coronary vascular disease (Patelaron 2012). The nutrient requirements of lactation are higher than during pregnancy. Table 6.1 includes the DRIs for breast-feeding women. These women should meet their own postpartum nutritional needs as well as produce an adequate volume of milk to meet their babies' nutritional needs.

## ENERGY

Among mothers exclusively breast-feeding their infants, the energy demands of lactation exceed prepregnancy demands by ~500 kcal/day for milk production of 780 ml/day for the first 6 months of lactation (Kitzmiller 2008). These needs may be partially met by extra fat stored during pregnancy (Table 6.8).

## Table 6.8 Energy Adjustments for Lactation

| Lactation | EER = prepregnancy EER + milk energy output − weight loss |
|---|---|
| First 6 months | EER + 500 − 170 kcal/day |
| Second 6 months | EER + 400 kcal/day − 0 |

EER = estimated energy requirements.

Adapted from Institute of Medicine Food and Nutrition Board: *Dietary Reference Intakes: The Essential Guide to Nutrient Requirements*. Washington, DC, The National Academies Press, 2006

Women should consume a minimum of 1,800 kcal/day. Individual energy needs vary depending on the volume of milk produced, the amount of stored fat, and the woman's energy expenditure (Reader 2004).

The relationship between breast-feeding and weight loss is neither consistent nor conclusive. Women who are breast-feeding should be given realistic, health-promoting advice about weight changes in lactation. Many women lose weight during the first 6 months of lactation, but some women maintain weight. The average rate of weight loss is ~0.5–1 kg/month (~1–2 lb/month) after the first month postpartum, with 1–2 kg/month (4–5 lb) acceptable for women who are overweight (Institute of Medicine 1991). Rapid weight loss (>2 kg/month [>4.4 lb/month] after the first month postpartum) is not advised for breast-feeding women. Intakes of <1,500 kcal/day have resulted in decreased milk output (Strode 1986). Extreme diets and weight-loss medications are not recommended.

## MACRONUTRIENTS

To meet the additional demand during lactation, the estimated average requirement (EAR) for carbohydrates is 160 g/day with an RDA of 210 g/day (Institute of Medicine Food and Nutrition Board 2006). This should be sufficient carbohydrate for an adequate volume of milk, to prevent ketonemia, and to maintain appropriate glucose levels during lactation (Reader 2004).

Fat intake approximates 20–35% of energy. The adequate intake for essential fatty acids is the same as during pregnancy, 13 g/day of omega-6 (n-6) fatty acids and 1.4 g/day of omega-3(n-3) fatty acids (National Research Council 2009). Inclusion of 8–12 oz of seafood per week is recommended, with the mercury concerns as reviewed earlier for pregnancy (American Diabetes Association 2008a, U.S. Department of Agriculture, Center for Nutrition Policy and Promotion 2012).

The RDA for protein in lactation is set to preserve muscle and maintain milk production. The EAR for protein is 1.05 g/kg/day with an RDA of 71 g/day (Institute of Medicine Food and Nutrition Board 2006, Reader 2004).

Breast-feeding mothers do not need to drink large amounts of fluids to produce sufficient milk; they should be advised to drink to thirst. Total water intake includes drinking water and other beverages, but also fluids as part of foods (~22%) (Kitzmiller 2008). The DRI for water in lactation is 13 cups/day or 9–10 cups of beverages. Encouraging mothers to sip on a beverage (preferably water or caffeine-free tea) while nursing, with a goal of keeping their urine a pale yellow color, may be a helpful guideline.

## MICRONUTRIENTS

Women with PDM should be encouraged to continue with a nutrient-dense diet through the course of lactation. During the postpartum period, the need for supplementation depends on the woman's nutritional status. Women found to be anemic after delivery or at their postpartum checkup should take 60–120 mg/day of elemental iron until the anemia is resolved. Although routine vitamin and mineral supplementation in lactating women is not recommended, specific nutrient supplementation may be warranted for women at nutritional risk.

Human milk alone cannot meet the vitamin D needs of the infant. It is recommended that all breast-fed infants receive 200 IU of oral vitamin D drops for the first 2 months of life and until daily consumption of vitamin D fortified milk or formula reaches 500 ml/day (Gartner 2005).

## ALCOHOL

Alcohol consumption while breast-feeding may have adverse effects on the infant's feeding as well as glucose control (Kitzmiller 2008).

Pregnant women without diabetes do not appear to experience significant changes between pre– and post–breast-feeding blood glucose, nor do they exhibit any hypoglycemic responses to lactation (Gartner 2005). Blood glucose, however, may be more variable during lactation for women with T1D, and both hyper- and hypoglycemia are possible. The extent of variability may depend on the amount of milk produced and the frequency of feeding (Bentley-Lewis 2007). Hypoglycemia is most likely to occur within 1 h after breast-feeding, so periodic SMBG at this time is encouraged to determine the need for, and timing of, snacks. Episodes of hypoglycemia may be avoided by eating a snack of a minimum of 15 g of carbohydrate and protein (Bradley 2007). The inclusion of a snack containing carbohydrate and protein before bed may avoid nighttime hypoglycemia (2:00–6:00 A.M.). Adjustments to evening insulin doses also can be made. Because most women experience fatigue postpartum and sleep more, there is a risk that they will sleep through a meal or snack, with resulting hypoglycemia. To avoid this, women should be encouraged to nap after meals and snacks, not before. Continuation of the pregnancy meal plan often is suggested, along with SBGM to meet the glycemic targets and assure adequate nutrition.

## COURSE OF LACTATION

Women with diabetes are at increased risk for lactation complications (Lawrence 2005). Poor metabolic control during pregnancy can negatively affect serum prolactin as well as placental lactogen and mammary development, which ultimately can affect milk production (Neubauer 1990). In addition, mothers with diabetes tend to have lower prolactin and higher nitrogen levels than nondiabetic mothers in the first week, which correlates with slower onset of copious milk production. Fluctuations in blood glucose levels after birth can impair lactose synthesis (Arthur 1994, Hartmann 2001, Oliveira 2008) and delay the onset of lactogenesis an average of 15–28 h (Arthur 1989). Glucose management during lactation can negatively affect milk production (Neubauer 1993), and lower infant intake has been observed, even in women with normal blood glucose levels (Miyake 1989). Concomitant thyroid dysfunction also may interfere with lactation (Marasco 2006).

Hypoglycemia, respiratory distress, or other complications in the infant of a mother with diabetes also can necessitate supplementation and interference with the early establishment of breast-feeding. Early and frequent feedings may help to minimize neonatal hypoglycemia, but mothers at risk may desire to manually express and freeze colostrum during the last trimester to use at the hospital if supplementation becomes necessary (Cox 2006). Although they have more difficulty in the beginning and have a higher fallout rate, nursing mothers with diabetes who make it past the early weeks have the same duration of breast-feeding as nondiabetic nursing mothers (Ferris 1993).

Women with diabetes are also more prone to mastitis and candidal infections of the nipple and breast during lactation (Arthur 1994). Optimal management of diabetes minimizes such complications, and with good metabolic control, nursing mothers who have diabetes breast-feed as well as their nonaffected counterparts once they successfully navigate any early postpartum issues (Ferris 1993, Stage 2006, American Dietetic Association 2009).

## SELECTED READINGS

Academy of Nutrition and Dietetics (formerly American Dietetic Association): *Medical Nutrition Therapy, Evidence-Based Guides for Practice: Gestational Diabetes Mellitus Evidence-Based Guide for Practice.* Chicago, American Dietetic Association, 2008

Academy of Nutrition and Dietetics (formerly American Dietetic Association): *Medical Nutrition Therapy, Evidence-Based Guides for Practice: Type 1 & 2 Diabetes Mellitus Evidence-Based Guide for Practice.* Chicago, American Dietetic Association, 2008

American Diabetes Association: Managing preexisting diabetes for pregnancy. Consensus statement. *Diabetes Care* 31:1060–1079, 2008

American Diabetes Association: Nutrition Recommendations and interventions for diabetes. Position statement. *Diabetes Care* 31 (Suppl. 1):S61–S68, 2008

American Dietetic Association: Nutrition and lifestyle for a healthy pregnancy outcome. Position statement. *J Am Diet Assoc* 108:553–560, 2008

American Dietetic Association: Position of the American Dietetic Association: Promoting and supporting breastfeeding. *J Am Diet Assoc* 109:1926–1942, 2009

California Department of Public Health: Prenatal weight gain grids. Available at http://www.cdph.ca.gov/pubsforms/forms/Pages/MaternalandChildHealth.aspx. Accessed 8 September 2012

California Diabetes and Pregnancy Program: *Sweet Success California Diabetes and Pregnancy Program Guidelines for Care.* Revised ed. Sacramento, CA, State of California Department of Public Health, Maternal, Child and Adolescent Health Division, 2008

Diabetes Care and Education Practice Group, American Dietetic Association: *On the Cutting Edge: Diabetes and Pregnancy* 28:2, 2007

Kitzmiller JL, Block JM, Brown FM, Conway DL, Coustan DR, Gunderson EP, Herman WH, Hoffman LD, Inturrisi M, Jovanovic LB, Kjos SI, Knopp RH, Montoro MN, Ogata ES, Paramsothy P, Reader DM, Rosenn BM, Thomas AM: *Management of Preexisting Diabetes and Pregnancy.* Alexandria, VA, American Diabetes Association, 2008

Lawrence RA, Lawrence RM: *Breastfeeding: A Guide for the Medical Profession.* 7th ed. Philadelphia, PA, Elsevier Mosby, 2011

Thomas A: Pregnancy with pre-existing diabetes. In *The Art and Science of Diabetes Self-Management Education. A Desk Reference for Healthcare Professionals.* Messing, C, Ed. Chicago, IL, American Association of Diabetes Educators, 2006

U.S. Department of Agriculture, Center for Nutrition Policy and Promotion: My plate daily meal plans for pregnancy and breastfeeding. Available at http://www.choosemyplate.gov/mypyramidmoms. Accessed 8 September 2012

U.S. Department of Agriculture, Center for Nutrition Policy and Promotion: *Report of the Dietary Guidelines Advisory Committee on the Dietary Guidelines for Americans, 2010.* Available at http://www.cnpp.usda.gov/dgas2010-dgacreport.htm. Accessed 24 March 2013

---

## REFERENCES

American Academy of Pediatrics, Section on Breastfeeding: Breastfeeding and the use of human milk. Policy statement. *Pediatrics* 115:496–506, 2005

American Beverage Association: Caffeine comparison. Available at http://www.ameribev.org/nutrition--science/beverage-ingredients/caffeine. Accessed 10 August 2012

American College of Obstetricians and Gynecologists: Anemia in pregnancy. Practice bulletin. *Obstet Gynecol* 112:201–207, 2008

American College of Obstetricians and Gynecologists: Obesity in pregnancy. Committee opinion no. 315. *Obstet Gynecol* 106:671–675, 2005

American Diabetes Association: Standards of medical care in diabetes—2013. *Diabetes Care* 36 (Suppl. 1):S11–S66, 2013

American Diabetes Association: National standards for diabetes self-management education. *Diabetes Care* 33 (Suppl. 1):S89–S96, 2010

American Diabetes Association: Managing preexisting diabetes for pregnancy. Consensus statement. *Diabetes Care* 31:1060–1079, 2008a

American Diabetes Association: Nutrition recommendations and interventions for diabetes. Position statement. *Diabetes Care* 31 (Suppl. 1):S61–S68, 2008b

American Diabetes Association: Gestational diabetes mellitus. *Diabetes Care* 27 (Suppl. 1):S88–S90, 2004

American Dietetic Association: Position of the American Dietetic Association: Promoting and supporting breastfeeding. *J Am Diet Assoc* 109:1926–1942, 2009

American Dietetic Association: Nutrition and lifestyle for a healthy pregnancy outcome. Position statement. *J Am Diet Assoc* 108:553–560, 2008

Arthur PG, Kent JC, Hartmann PE: Metabolites of lactose synthesis in milk from diabetic and nondiabetic women during lactogenesis II. *J Pediatr Gastroenterol Nutr* 19:100–108, 1994

Arthur PG, Smith M, Hartmann PE: Milk lactose, citrate, and glucose as markers of lactogenesis in normal and diabetic women. *J Pediatr Gastroenterol Nutr* 9:488–496, 1989

Barker M, Brand-Miller JC, Moses RG, Petocz P, Winter M: Can a low glycemic diet reduce the need for insulin in gestational diabetes mellitus? *Diabetes Care* 32:996–1000, 2009

Bentley-Lewis R, Goldfine AB, Green DE, Seely EW: Lactation after normal pregnancy is not associated with blood glucose fluctuations. *Diabetes Care* 30:2792–2793, 2007

Bradley C: Managing diabetes while breast-feeding. *Diabetes Self Manag* 24:84, 87–89, 2007

Cox S: Expressing and storing colostrum antenatally for use in the newborn period. *Breastfeeding Review* 14:5–8, 2006

Crume TL, Ogden L, Maligie MB, Sheffield S, Bischoff K, McDuffie R, Daniels S, Hamman RF, Norris JM, Dabelea D: Long-term impact of neonatal breast-feeding on childhood adiposity and fat distribution among children exposed to diabetes in utero. *Diabetes Care* 34:641–645, 2011

Dennedy MC, Avalos G, O'Reilly MW, O'Sullivan EP, Gaffney G, Dunne F: Atlantic-DIP: raised maternal body mass index (BMI) adversely affects maternal and fetal outcomes in glucose-tolerant women according to the International Association of Diabetes and Pregnancy Study Group. *J Clin Endocrin Metab* 97:E608–E612, 2012

Dornhurst A, Nicholls JSD, Probst F, Patterson CM, Hollier KL, Elkeles RS, Beard RW: Calorie restriction for the treatment of gestational diabetes. *Diabetes* 40:161–164, 1991

EnergyFiend: Caffeine content of drinks and products. Available at http://www.energyfiend.com/the-caffeine-database. Accessed 10 August 2012

Ferris AM, Neubauer SH, Bendel RB, Green KW, Ingardia CJ, Reece EA: Perinatal lactation protocol and outcome in mothers with and without insulin-dependent diabetes mellitus. *Am J Clin Nutr* 58:43–48, 1993

Gartner LM, Morton J, Lawrence RA, Naylor AJ, O'Hare D, Schanler RJ, Eidleman AI: American Academy of Pediatrics, Section on Breastfeeding: Breast-feeding and the use of human milk. Policy statement. *Pediatrics* 115:496–506, 2005

Hartmann P, Cregan M: Lactogenesis and the effects of insulin-dependent diabetes mellitus and prematurity. *J Nutr* 131:3016S–3020S, 2001

Higdon JV, Frei B: Coffee and health: a review of recent human research. *Crit Rev Food Sci Nutr* 46:101–123, 2006

Hummel S, Pfluger M, Kriechauf S, Hummel M, Ziegler AG: Predictors of over-weight during childhood in offspring of parents with type 1 diabetes. *Diabetes Care* 32:921–925, 2009

Institute of Medicine: *Nutrition During Lactation.* Washington, DC, The National Academies Press, 1991.

Institute of Medicine, National Research Council: *Weight Gain During Pregnancy: Reexamining the Guidelines.* Rasmussen KM, Taktine AL, Eds. Washington, DC, The National Academies Press, 2009

Institute of Medicine, Food and Nutrition Board: *Dietary Reference Intakes for Calcium and Vitamin D.* Washington, DC, The National Academies Press, 2010

Institute of Medicine, Food and Nutrition Board: *Dietary Reference Intakes: The Essential Guide to Nutrient Requirements.* Washington, DC, The National Academies Press, 2006

Institute of Medicine, Food and Nutrition Board: *Dietary Reference Intakes for Vitamin A, Vitamin K, Arsenic, Boron, Chromium, Copper, Iodine, Iron, Manganese, Molybenum, Nickle, Silicon, Vanadium and Zinc.* Washington, DC, The National Academies Press, 2001

Institute of Medicine, Food and Nutrition Board: *National Academy of Sciences (US). Nutrition During Pregnancy: Weight Gain and Nutrient Supplements. Report of the Committee on Nutritional Status During Pregnancy and Lactation.* Washington, DC, The National Academies Press, 1990

Johnstone FD, Lindsay RS, Steel J: Type 1 diabetes and pregnancy: trends in birth weight over 40 years at a single clinic. *Obstet Gynec* 107:1297–1302, 2006

Jovanovic L, Knopp RH, Kim H, Cefalu WT, Zhu X-D, Lee YJ, Simpson JL, Mills JL: For the Diabetes in Early Pregnancy Study Group: elevated pregnancy losses at high and low extremes of maternal glucose in early normal and diabetic pregnancy. Evidence for a protective adaptation in diabetes. *Diabetes Care* 28:1113–1117, 2005

Kitzmiller JL, Block, JM, Brown FM, Conway DL, Coustan DR, Gunderson EP, Herman WH, Hoffman LD, Inturrisi M, Jovanovic LB, Kjos SI, Knopp RH, Montoro MN, Ogata ES, Paramsothy P, Reader DM, Rosenn BM, Thomas AM: *Management of Preexisting Diabetes and Pregnancy.* Alexandria, VA, American Diabetes Association, 2008

Knip N, Virtanen SM, Becker D, Dupre J, Krischer JP, Akerblom HK; TRIGR Study Group: Early feeding and risk of type 1 diabetes: experiences from the Trial to Reduce Insulin dependent diabetes mellitus in the Genetically at Risk (TRIGR). *Am J Clin Nutr* 94:1814S–1820S, 2011

Knopp RH, Magee MS, Raisys V, Benedetti TJ: Metabolic effects of hypocaloric diets in management of gestational diabetes. *Diabetes* 40:165–171, 1991

Lawrence RA, Lawrence RM: *Breastfeeding: A Guide for the Medical Profession.* 6th ed. Philadelphia, PA, Elsevier Mosby, 2005

Louie JCY, Markovic TP, Perera N, Foote P, Foote D, Petocz P, Ross JC, Brand-Miller JC: A randomized controlled trial investigating the effects of a low-glycemic index diet on pregnancy outcomes in gestational diabetes mellitus. *Diabetes Care* 34:2341–2346, 2011

Marasco L: The impact of thyroid dysfunction on lactation. *Breastfeeding Abstracts* 25:9, 11–12, 2006

Miyake A, Tahara M, Koike K, Tanizawa O: Decrease in neonatal suckled milk volume in diabetic women. *Eur J Obstet Gynecol Reprod Biol* 33:49–53, 1989

Murtaugh MA, Ferris AM, Capacchione CM, Reece EA: Energy intake and glycemia in lactating women with type 1 diabetes. *J Am Diet Assoc* 98:642–648, 1998

Neubauer SH: Lactation in insulin-dependent diabetes. *Prog Food Nutr Sci* 14:333–370, 1990

Neubauer SH, Ferris AM, Chase CG, Fanelli J, Thompson CA, Lammi-Keefe CJ, Clark RM, Jensen RG, Bendel RB, Green KW: Delayed lactogenesis in women with insulin-dependent diabetes mellitus. *Am J Clin Nutr* 58:54–60, 1993

Oliveira AM, da Cunha CC, Penha-Silva N, Abdallah VO, Jorge PT: [Interference of the blood glucose control in the transition between phases I and II of lactogenesis in patients with type 1 diabetes mellitus]. *Arq Bras Endocrinol Metabol* 52:473–481, 2008

Patelarou E, Girvalaki C, Brokalaki H, Patelarou A, Androulaki Z, Vardavas C: Current evidence on the associations of breastfeeding, infant formula, and cow's milk introduction with type 1 diabetes mellitus: a systematic review. *Nutr Rev* 70:509–519, 2012

Reader D, Franz MJ: Lactation, diabetes and nutrition recommendations. *Curr Diabetes Rep* 4:370–376, 2004

Reader D, Splett P, Gunderson E: Impact of gestational diabetes mellitus nutrition practice guidelines implemented by registered dietitians on pregnancy outcome. *J Am Diet Assoc* 106:1426–1433, 2006

Sparud-Lundin C, Wennergren N, Elfvin A, Berg M: Breastfeeding in women with type 1 diabetes: exploration of predictive factors. *Diabetes Care* 34:296–301, 2011

Stage E, Norgard H, Damm P, Mathiesen E: Long-term breast-feeding in women with type 1 diabetes. *Diabetes Care* 29:771–774, 2006

Strode MA, Dewey KG, Lonnerdal B: Effects of short-term caloric restriction on lactational performance of well-nourished women. *Acta Paediatr Scand* 75:222–229, 1986

U.S. Department of Agriculture, Center for Nutrition Policy and Promotion: *Report of the Dietary Guidelines Advisory Committee on the Dietary Guidelines for*

*Americans, 2010.* Available at http://www.fns.usda.gov/dietaryguidelines. Accessed 10 August 2012

U.S. Department of Agriculture, Food Safety: Food safety for pregnant women, 2006 (slightly revised 2011). Available at http://www.fda.gov/Food/Resources-ForYou/Consumers/SelectedHealthTopics/ucm312704.htm. Accessed 28 August 2012

Wheeler ML, Pi-Sunyer FX: Carbohydrate issues: type and amount. *J Am Diet Assoc* 108:S34–S39, 2008

# Use of Insulin During Pregnancy in Preexisting Diabetes

# Highlights
## Use of Insulin During Pregnancy in Preexisting Diabetes

■ The metabolic alterations in early pregnancy include loss of glucose and gluconeogenic substrates, which can lead to hypoglycemia, especially during the night.

■ During midgestation, insulin requirements begin to increase as the woman changes to a lipid-based energy economy.

■ In late gestation, insulin resistance due to placental production of contrainsulin hormones results in even greater insulin requirements.

■ Insulin injections may not be necessary during the immediate postpartum period because of the rapid decrease in insulin resistance after delivery of the fetus and placenta. Insulin need requires recalculation using postpartum weight and plans for diet, exercise, and breast-feeding.

■ To deal with these metabolic changes and maintain normal blood glucose levels, the pregnant diabetic woman must perform frequent self-monitoring of blood glucose, and she and her health-care team must be equipped to make dosage adjustments in response to trends in blood glucose values.

■ A multiple-injection routine is necessary to replicate normal meal-stimulated insulin output during pregnancy. The use of insulin pumps may be appropriate.

■ During active labor, when insulin requirements disappear and glucose requirements remain relatively constant, target glucose levels of 70–90 mg/dl (3.9–5.0 mmol/l) should be maintained.

# Use of Insulin During Pregnancy in Preexisting Diabetes

## METABOLIC ALTERATIONS DURING NORMAL GESTATION

During normal pregnancy, metabolism adapts to meet maternal needs and provide fuel for the growing fetoplacental unit (Freinkel 1980). Beginning in early gestation, glucose reaches the fetus by facilitated diffusion—it crosses the placenta at a rate faster than would be predicted physiologically. Similarly, amino acids are transported actively to the fetal circulation against a concentration gradient. Of particular importance is a decrease in the maternal plasma concentration of the gluconeogenic amino acid alanine.

Transfer of glucose and gluconeogenic substrate to the fetus occurs concomitantly and conspires to cause maternal hypoglycemia during early pregnancy. Toward the end of the first trimester, it is common for insulin requirements in women with type 1 diabetes (T1D) to diminish by 10–20% of the dosage taken before conception (Garcia-Patterson 2010). Moreover, blood glucose control during the first trimester is more unstable than usual, and nocturnal hypoglycemia is especially common.

At 16–24 weeks of gestation, the so-called diabetogenic stress of pregnancy begins, and daily insulin requirement typically begins to increase (Garcia-Patterson 2010). At this time, the mother switches from a primarily glucose-based to a lipid-based energy economy derived from either circulating fats or stored adipose tissue to spare glucose for fetal growth.

In late pregnancy, basal insulin levels are higher than normal nongravid levels, and eating produces a two- to threefold greater outpouring of insulin (insulin requirement is usually 0.9–1.2 units/kg/24 h [0.4–0.6 units/lb/24 h]). These increases in plasma insulin are opposed by diminished responsiveness to insulin action because of placental production of contrainsulin hormones—human placental lactogen, prolactin, estrogen, and progesterone—and increased maternal production of cortisol.

During the second and third trimesters, insulin requirements gradually increase to as much as twice the total daily dosage of insulin needed before pregnancy. Placental growth and the production of contrainsulin hormones plateau at ~36 weeks. As a result, the dosage of insulin necessary to maintain euglycemia peaks at 37 weeks (Garcia-Patterson 2010). A decrease in insulin requirement after 37 weeks should not necessarily be interpreted as an indication of a failing fetoplacental unit.

After delivery of the placenta, human placental lactogen, estrogen, and progesterone rapidly clear from the circulation, leading to a marked decrease in insulin resistance. Pituitary growth hormone and gonadotropin remain suppressed, despite the falling placental hormones. The result is a state of "panhypopituitarism." In addition, high prepartum doses of insulin create stores of bound insulin that continue to be released. Therefore, it is sometimes unnecessary to resume subcutaneous insulin injections during the immediate postpartum period. The dosage of insulin required postpartum must be recalculated based on postpartum weight, diet, exercise, and plans for breast-feeding.

Understanding the marked metabolic alterations in normal pregnancies and pregnancies complicated by diabetes leads to several important clinical generalizations:

- Hyperglycemia exerts potentially devastating effects on the fetus throughout pregnancy and therefore must be avoided.
- Nongravid criteria cannot be used to assess metabolism during pregnancy. Therefore, separate standards must be used to monitor diabetes management (Freinkel 1990).
- Women with T1D require frequent (four to eight times per day) self-monitoring of blood glucose (SMBG) throughout gestation to promptly recognize the need for adjustments of their insulin dosage.
- Multiple injections of insulin are necessary to truly replicate the qualitative and quantitative changes in normal meal-related insulin output.

## THERAPEUTIC INSULIN USE

The primary goal of insulin replacement is to achieve plasma glucose concentrations nearly identical to those observed in nondiabetic women. The goal of rigid glycemic control, however, should not be maintained at the cost of symptomatic hypoglycemia. Insulin type and injection frequency must be individualized and the changing insulin requirements at various stages of gestation should be anticipated.

## INSULIN REGIMENS

Human insulins are the least immunogenic of all insulins. Various insulin preparations may be used in combination to achieve optimal glycemic control. The proper use of insulin requires an understanding of the factors that affect its absorption, disposal, and action. Table 7.1 lists the onset, peak, and duration of action of the most commonly used types of insulin.

A single daily injection of intermediate-acting (neutral protamine Hagedorn [NPH]) and short-acting (regular) insulin usually does not provide adequate insulin replacement to ensure satisfactory 24-h glycemic control. Most women with T1D require three or more daily injections (Jovanovic 1982, Hare 1989). Safe, rapid-acting insulins are now available that more closely mimic normal physiologic release of insulin compared with regular insulin, and there are also two basal insulin analogs, glargine and detemir, in addition to NPH. The optimal injection schedule during pregnancy has not been established, and currently many insulin regimens can be used to achieve glycemic control.

## Table 7.1 Insulins by Comparative Action

| | Onset (h) | Peak (h) | Effective duration (h) |
|---|---|---|---|
| **Rapid-acting [manufacturer-brand name]** | | | |
| Insulin lispro (analog) [Lilly-Humalog] | <0.25–0.5 | 0.5–2.5 | 3–5 |
| Insulin aspart (analog) [Novo Nordisk-Novolog] | <0.25 | 1–3 | 3–5 |
| Insulin glulisine (analog) [Sanofi Aventis-Apidra] | <0.25 | 0.75–2 | 3–5 |
| **Short-acting** | | | |
| Regular (soluble) [Lilly, Novo Nordisk] | 0.5–1 | 2–3 | 5–8 |
| U500R (concentrated) [Lilly]* | 0.5–1 | 2–3 | 18–24 |
| **Intermediate-acting** | | | |
| NPH (isophane) [Lilly, Novo Nordisk] | 2–4 | 4–10 | 10–16 |
| **Long-acting** | | | |
| Insulin glargine (analog) [Sanofi Aventis-Lantus] | 2 | Relatively flat | 11–24 |
| Insulin detemir (analog) [Novo Nordisk-Levemir] | 1–2 (dose dependent) | Relatively flat | Dose dependent; 12 h for 0.2 U/kg; 14 h for 0.4 U/kg, 7.6- 24 h Binds to albumin. |
| **Combinations** | | | |
| 70% NPH, 30% regular [Lilly] | 0.5–1 | Dual | 10–16 |
| 75% NPL, 25% lispro [Lilly] | <0.25 | Dual | 10–16 |
| 50% NPL, 50% lispro [Lilly] | <0.25 | Dual | 10–16 |
| 70% aspart protamine, 30% aspart [Novo Nordisk] | <0.25 | Dual | 15–24 |

* May be useful when total insulin dosage is >100 units at a time (which would ordinarily necessitate two injections); has similar onset and peak to regular insulin but longer duration.

NPH = neutral protamine Hagedorn.

A two-injection regimen may cause nocturnal hypoglycemic episodes if the intermediate-acting insulin given before the evening meal exerts its peak action during the middle of the night, especially in women with T1D. Fitful sleep, profuse sweating, nightmares, or morning headaches suggest nocturnal hypoglycemia. To eliminate the problem of nocturnal hypoglycemia, the evening dose of intermediate-acting insulin should be delayed until bedtime so that its peak action coincides with breakfast the next morning. Note that fasting hyperglycemia may signify a middle-of-the-night low. Women should perform SMBG with any symptom of hypoglycemia and may be asked to set an alarm clock to perform SMBG at 2:00 or 3:00 a.m. to rule out nocturnal hypoglycemia causing fasting hyperglycemia. In any regimen that includes a morning dose of rapid- and intermediate-acting insulins, lunch must be constant in composition and timing. Premixed insulins should be avoided as doses cannot be adjusted independently.

Greater precision of insulin administration and more flexibility can be achieved with multiple insulin injections. Rapid-acting insulin before each meal provides a degree of meal flexibility that may be advantageous for pregnant women. Intermediate-acting insulin, given twice daily or every 8 h, or a long-acting insulin analog, given once or twice daily, mimics the physiological secretion of basal insulin. These programs permit frequent adjustment of rapid-acting insulin to prevent hypoglycemia, particularly during the first trimester, when nausea and anorexia may be common. Patients must frequently perform SMBG and learn to anticipate insulin needs based on the carbohydrate content of the upcoming meal, the preprandial blood glucose, and the anticipated level of exercise. Generally, blood glucose should be measured four times (fasting and 1 or 2 h after each meal) to eight times (before and after each meal, at bedtime, and in the middle of the night) daily. Blood glucose also should be tested with any symptoms of hypoglycemia and before driving a vehicle.

Two rapid-acting insulin analogs, insulin lispro and insulin aspart, are Food and Drug Administration (FDA) Pregnancy Category B and are considered safe to use during pregnancy (Mathiesen 2011). To date, there are no clinical trials showing the safety and efficacy of insulin glulisine in pregnancy, and it is FDA pregnancy Category C.

There are two basal analogs, insulin glargine (SanofiAventis-Lantus) and insulin detemir (NovoNordisk-Levemir). The FDA recently changed the classification of insulin detemir to Pregnancy Category B based on the results of a multinational, randomized controlled trial (RCT) of 310 pregnant women with T1D that showed no difference in the incidence of adverse maternal or fetal outcomes in women using insulin detemir compared with women using NPH (Mathiesen 2012).

Insulin glargine is FDA Pregnancy Category C. Two meta-analyses of retrospective and case control studies did not show any difference in maternal (Lepercq 2012) or fetal (Pollex 2011, Lepercq 2012) outcomes. A transplacental transfer study (Pollex 2010) showed that insulin glargine is not likely to cross the placenta when used at therapeutic doses.

If insulin therapy is initiated during pregnancy, dosage can be calculated using the formula in Table 7.2

## INSULIN PUMPS

On the premise that the ultimate glycemic control is to mimic normal pancreatic insulin release, some clinicians prefer continuous subcutaneous insulin infusion via an insulin pump. Insulin pumps deliver a basal rate of rapid-acting insulin with pulse-dose increments before meals based on premeal glucose value and anticipated intake of carbohydrate. They have been used safely and successfully during pregnancy. Many women prefer an insulin pump as it may provide more

## Table 7.2 Insulin Starting Dosage Regimen for Diabetic Pregnancy

**NPH plus rapid-acting insulin schedule**

Patient's current weight in kg =_____ ,

| Gestational age (weeks) | 0–12 | 13–28 | 29–34 | 35–40 |
|---|---|---|---|---|
| Insulin dose | 0.7 unit | 0.8 unit | 0.9 unit | 1.0 unit |

Total Daily Dose (TDD) = weight in kg × desired units of insulin
Give 2/3 TDD prebreakfast; 1/3 TDD predinner
Divide prebreakfast dose into 2/3 NPH and 1/3 rapid-acting insulin
Divide predinner dose into 1/2 NPH and 1/2 rapid-acting insulin or give rapid-acting insulin predinner and NPH at bedtime

**Basal-bolus schedule**

Calculate TDD as above
Give 1/2 as basal insulin in one dose or split equally into 2 doses
Give 1/2 as bolus insulin split equally into 3 doses before each meal
Alternatively, bolus insulin may be given as 30% at breakfast, 25% at lunch, 25% at dinner and the remaining 15–20% given with snacks (Gabbe 2007)

NPH = neutral protamine Hagedorn.

flexibility in timing and composition of meals. A meta-analysis of RCTs comparing women treated with multiple daily injections (MDI) to women treated with continuous subcutaneous insulin infusion (CSII) showed no significant difference in pregnancy outcomes and glycemic control (Mukhopadhyay 2007).

The basal infusion rate is usually ~50–60% of the total daily dose of insulin. Many women will require at least three infusion rates: midnight to 4:00 a.m., 4:00 a.m. to 10:00 a.m., 10:00 a.m. to midnight. The lowest basal dose is usually administered at midnight to 4:00 a.m. and will help prevent nocturnal hypoglycemia. From 4:00 a.m. to 10:00 a.m., cortisol and growth hormone levels rise, and the basal rate of insulin must be increased. The progressive increase in contrainsulin hormones accompanying pregnancy will require a corresponding increase in basal infusion rates, meal boluses, and insulin sensitivity factor. If the basal infusion rates are calculated properly, glucose concentrations will be within target before meals, and each meal or snack will require a bolus of insulin. The remaining 40–50% of the total daily dose of insulin is given as meal boluses. Fixed boluses may be used with 30% given at breakfast, 25% at lunch, 25% at dinner, and the remaining 15–20% given with snacks (Gabbe 2007). Alternately, a woman can use a carbohydrate ratio, where the pump is programmed to give 1 unit of insulin for a given amount of carbohydrates (e.g., 1 unit:10 g carbohydrate). The disadvantages of insulin pump therapy are the cost of an insulin pump and supplies and the potential for hyperglycemia and diabetic ketoacidosis to develop rapidly if there is pump failure.

## DOSAGE ADJUSTMENT

Patients are encouraged to check blood glucose levels frequently and record the results in a form that permits recognition of glycemic patterns. The essential principles for any successful insulin regimen include observation of glucose patterns and gradual (usually 10–20%) prospective dosage adjustments.

For example, a patient experiencing elevated blood glucose concentrations during the late afternoon should not react by giving supplemental insulin before dinner and risking hypoglycemia later in the evening. Instead, she should plan to increase her morning dose of intermediate-acting insulin the next morning (if she is taking a mixed morning dose) or to increase her noon dose of rapid-acting insulin. In another case, a woman with satisfactory fasting blood glucose but low mid-morning value would reduce the morning dose of rapid-acting insulin. There are exceptions, however. For example, a hypoglycemic reaction that is followed by an elevated blood glucose value does not necessarily warrant a change in dosage. Instead, possible explanations for the hypoglycemic episode should be explored and corrected. Adjustments can be made to correct preprandial hypo- or hyperglycemia using an insulin sensitivity factor (ISF) or "correction factor," such as 1 unit-to-50 mg/dl. Using this correction factor, a woman would take 1 unit less rapid-acting insulin with her meal if her blood glucose value was below 50 mg/dl or take an extra unit if her blood glucose value is 150 mg/dl. This correction factor also could be used to correct postprandial hyperglycemia, but the duration of insulin action must be taken into account. Rapid-acting insulins have a duration of 3–5 h, so taking a "correction" dose 2 h after a meal may lead to hypoglycemia later on. It is expected that insulin doses will rise as the pregnancy progresses.

## INSULIN USE FOR PRETERM DELIVERY

Preterm delivery can be particularly hazardous and presents a special therapeutic dilemma in diabetic pregnancy (see also chapter on neonatal care). β-Sympathomimetics, such as terbutaline and ritodrine, are capable of causing rapid and extreme elevations in maternal glucose concentration and possibly ketoacidosis and should be avoided in women with diabetes. Magnesium sulfate, although not very effective as a tocolytic agent, is prescribed just before birth to patients expected to deliver prior to 32 weeks' gestation to lessen the likelihood of cerebral palsy in the premature neonate (American College of Obstetricians and Gynecologists 2010). Indomethacin or calcium channel blockers may be used for tocolysis in women with diabetes. Tocolytic therapy should be undertaken only in centers in which continuous, experienced maternal–fetal supervision is available. Throughout parenteral tocolytic therapy, maternal glucose levels initially should be measured hourly and every 2–4 h once blood glucose is stable. Intravenous (IV) insulin should be administered as necessary.

Corticosteroids, used to accelerate fetal lung maturation, can further exacerbate hyperglycemia. If preterm labor results in preterm delivery, however, respiratory distress syndrome in the premature infant is more likely to result when steroids have not been administered. The usual dose of corticosteroids is two doses of β-methasone 12 mg given intramuscularly (IM) 24 h apart or four doses of dexamethasone 6 mg given IM 12 h apart. Blood glucose concentrations should be checked frequently, and supplemental rapid-acting insulin should be given as needed or short-acting insulin given as a continuous IV infusion during cortico-steroid administration and for several days afterward.

## INSULIN DURING LABOR AND DELIVERY

Intrapartum glycemic control plays a major role in the well-being of the neonate. Maternal hyperglycemia during labor may be associated with fetal acidemia, and is a major cause of neonatal hypoglycemia. At the onset of active labor, insulin requirements decrease, and glucose requirements are relatively constant at ~2.5 mg/kg/min (1.1 mg/lb/min) (Jovanovic 1983, 2004). From these data, Jovanovic and Peterson developed a protocol for meeting the glucose needs of active labor. The goal is to maintain a plasma glucose concentration between 70 and 90 mg/dl (3.9 and 5.0 mmol/l). A woman with an insulin pump may be allowed to continue her pump during labor, adjusting basal rates as needed. Alternatively, the pump may be discontinued and the following approach utilizing IV insulin may be utilized for more rapid control if glucose exceeds or dips below goals.

### MANAGEMENT FOR PLANNED INDUCTION:

- On the evening before elective induction, the usual bedtime dose of inter-mediate-acting insulin may be given.
- On the morning of induction, insulin is withheld and an IV infusion of normal saline or 5% dextrose in half-normal saline at 100–125 ml/h (to provide for energy requirements) is begun.
- Once active labor commences or plasma glucose level falls to <70 mg/dl (<3.9 mmol/l), normal saline should be changed to 5% dextrose in half-normal saline, and infused at a rate of 100–125 ml/min.
- Glucose level should be monitored hourly, and if it is <60 mg/dl (<3.3 mmol/l), the infusion rate should be doubled for the subsequent hour.
- If the plasma glucose concentration rises to >120 mg/dl (>6.7 mmol/l), an infusion of short-acting insulin in normal saline should be added by pig-gyback into the dextrose-containing IV. The concentration of insulin in the normal saline can be varied to avoid fluid overload. An example of the start-ing point would be 25 units of insulin in 250 ml of saline with an infusion rate of 10 ml/h through an infusion pump.
- Before epidural anesthesia, when rapid IV hydration is desired to avoid hypotension, non–glucose-containing fluids should be used because rapid IV glucose infusion can cause fetal acidemia.

### WHEN ELECTIVE CESAREAN DELIVERY IS PLANNED:

- The bedtime dose of intermediate-acting insulin may be given the night before surgery and surgery should be scheduled for early morning.
- The woman is instructed to take nothing by mouth (NPO) after midnight and the morning insulin is not given the day of surgery.

■ If surgery is later in the day, one-third to one-half of the woman's intermediate-acting dose of insulin may be given on the morning of surgery and every 8 h if surgery is delayed.
■ A dextrose infusion as described previously may be started if the glucose concentration falls to <60 mg/dl (<3.3 mmol/l).
■ Alternatively, glycemic control before elective cesarean delivery can be achieved with an infusion of 1–2 units/h IV regular insulin given simultaneously with 5 g/h dextrose. The insulin infusion should be discontinued immediately before surgery.
■ Hourly blood glucose determinations are recommended to allow for individualization of these protocols.

## POSTPARTUM INSULIN REQUIREMENTS

After delivery, insulin requirements diminish precipitously. As a result, it is often unnecessary to administer subcutaneous insulin for 1 or more days, particularly when patients are not eating after a cesarean section. Insulin requirements should be recalculated at 0.6 unit/kg/24 h (2.7 unit/lb/24 h), based on postpartum weight and should be started when either postprandial or fasting glucose is >150 mg/dl (>8.3 mmol/l). The prepregnancy dose may be resumed if it is known or one-third to one-half of the end-of-pregnancy dose can be given. Similar adjustments are made in women on insulin pump therapy.

## BREAST-FEEDING

There are few data on the changes in insulin requirements necessary to maintain good metabolic control while breast-feeding. Less insulin may be required during lactation and glucose control may be erratic. Episodes of hypoglycemia may be common, so glucose levels should be monitored frequently. Recommendations for lactating mothers include increasing calorie intake while maintaining the decreased postpartum insulin dosage (see chapter on nutritional management).

The optimal insulin program varies for each patient, and SMBG should provide the data necessary to adjust the dosage and timing of insulin injections. Because hypoglycemia is most likely to occur within an hour after breast-feeding, this is an important time to measure blood glucose. In most cases, hypoglycemia can be avoided by eating a small snack before breast-feeding rather than making frequent adjustments of the insulin dosage. Nocturnal hypoglycemia is particularly common. Therefore, blood glucose should be checked periodically during the night, and the evening dose of intermediate-acting insulin should be decreased if hypoglycemia is documented (Inturrisi 2008).

## ORAL ANTIDIABETES AGENTS

In the U.S., oral antidiabetes agents generally are not recommended for use by individuals with preexisting diabetes during pregnancy. Although there are no published controlled studies, isolated reports of human teratogenesis exist. Some of these agents have been recommended for use by patients with gestational diabetes, but no long-term follow-up studies on the offspring have been carried out, and no study to date has shown that they are safe or efficacious in the treatment of preexisting diabetes in pregnancy.

Sulfonylureas cross the placenta (Hebert 2009) and would be expected to increase fetal insulin production. Because hyperinsulinism contributes to abnormal fetal growth, use of these drugs is at least theoretically inappropriate. Metformin freely crosses the placenta (Vanky 2005), and few human or animal studies have evaluated potential beneficial or harmful effects.

## REFERENCES

American College of Obstetricians and Gynecologists: Magnesium sulfate before anticipated preterm birth for neuroprotection. Committee Opinion No. 455. *Obstet Gynecol* 115:669–671, 2010

Freinkel N: Banting Lecture 1980: of pregnancy and progeny. *Diabetes* 29:1023–1035, 1980

Freinkel N, Phelps R, Metzger BE: The mother in pregnancies complicated by diabetes. In *Diabetes Mellitus. Theory and Practice.* 4th ed. Rifkin H, Porte D Jr, Eds. New York, NY, Elsevier, 1990, p. 634–650

Gabbe SG, Carpenter LB, Garrison EA: New strategies for glucose control in patients with type 1 and type 2 diabetes mellitus in pregnancy. *Clin Obs & Gyn* 50:1014–1024, 2007

Garcia-Patterson A, Gich I, Amini SB, Catalano PM, deLeiva A, Corcoy R: Insulin requirements throughout pregnancy in women with type 1 diabetes mellitus: three changes of direction. *Diabetologia* 53:446–451, 2010

Hare JW: *Diabetes Complicating Pregnancy: The Joslin Clinic Method.* New York, NY, Liss, 1989

Hebert MF, Ma X, Naraharisetti SB, et al.: Are we optimizing gestational diabetes treatment with glyburide? The pharmacologic basis for better clinical practice. *Clin Pharmacol Ther* 85:607–614, 2009

Inturrisi M, Thomas A, Block JM, Kitzmiller JL: Breast-feeding and diabetes. In *Managing Preexisting Diabetes and Pregnancy: Technical Reviews and Consensus Recommendations for Care.* Kitzmiller JL, Jovanovic L, Brown F, Coustan DR, Reader DM, Eds. Alexandria, VA, American Diabetes Association, 2008, p. 697–727

Jovanovic L: Glucose and insulin requirements during labor and delivery: the case for normoglycemia in pregnancies complicated by diabetes. *Endocr Pract* 10:40–45, 2004

Jovanovic L, Peterson CM: Insulin and glucose requirements during the first stage of labor in insulin-dependent diabetic women. *Am J Med* 75:607–612, 1983

Jovanovic L, Peterson CM: Optimal insulin delivery for the pregnant diabetic patient. *Diabetes Care* 5 (Suppl. 1):S24–S35, 1982

Lepercq J, Lin J, Hall GC, Wang E, Dain MP, Riddle MC, Home PD: Meta-analysis of maternal and neonatal outcomes associated with the use of insulin glargine versus NPH insulin during pregnancy. *Obstet Gynecol International* 2012; epublished 16 May 2012 doi: 10.1155/2012/649070

Mathiesen ER, Damm P, Jovanovic L, McCance DR, Thyregod C, Jensen AB: Basal insulin analogues in diabetic pregnancy: a literature review and baseline results of a randomized, controlled trial in type 1 diabetes. *Diabetes Metab Res Rev* 27:543–551, 2011

Mathiesen ER, Hod M, Ivanisevic M, et al., on behalf of the Detemir in Pregnancy Study Group: Maternal efficacy and safety outcomes in a randomized, controlled trial comparing insulin detemir with NPH insulin in 310 pregnant women with type 1 diabetes. *Diabetes Care* 2012; epublished 30 July 2012 doi:10.2337/dc11-22645

Mukhopadhyay A, Farrell T, Fraser RB, Ola B: Continuous subcutaneous insulin infusion vs intensive conventional insulin therapy in pregnant diabetic women: a systematic review and metaanalysis of randomized, controlled trials. *Am J Obstet Gynecol* 197:447–456, 2007

Pollex E, Moretti ME, Koren G, Feig D: Safety of insulin glargine use in pregnancy: a systematic review and meta-analysis. *Ann Pharmacother* 45:9–16, 2011

Pollex EK, Feig DS, Lubetsky A, Yip PM, Koren G: Insulin glargine safety in pregnancy: a transplacental transfer study. *Diab Care* 33:29–33, 2010

Vanky E, Zahlsen K, Spigset O, Carlsen SM. Placental passage of metformin in women with polycystic ovary syndrome. *Fertil Steril* 83:1575–1578, 2005

# Diagnostic Testing and Fetal Surveillance

# Highlights
## Diagnostic Testing and Fetal Surveillance

■ Ultrasound is useful in determining gestational age, evaluating fetal anatomy, assessing fetal growth and weight, and determining fetal well-being during an antepartum biophysical profile.

■ Maternal serum α-fetoprotein and multiple marker screening can determine open fetal defects and some aneuploidies near 16 weeks of gestation.

■ Genetic tests, such as amniocentesis and chorionic villus sampling, can be used to detect many inherited disorders, so genetic counseling enables the determination of which disorders the tests should examine.

■ Antepartum fetal status can be determined through the evaluation of the fetal heart rate pattern. Antepartum tests have reduced the necessity for preterm delivery of infants of mothers with diabetes.

■ The use of tocolytic agents to suppress preterm labor in women with diabetes, and corticosteroids to accelerate lung maturation of the fetus, should be accompanied by careful attention to maternal metabolism since these agents may cause hyperglycemia.

# Diagnostic Testing and Fetal Surveillance

D iagnostic testing and fetal surveillance include various forms of testing performed during pregnancy to assess the normalcy and development of the
fetus (Table 8.1). Each mode of testing is described in the order in which it
usually is applied as pregnancy progresses. It is important that both caregivers and
patients understand that no test exists that can ensure the birth of a perfectly normal baby. One can only look for known problems with specific tests. Therefore, no
assurance can be made that "everything will be fine," no matter how many normal
test results are reported.

## DIAGNOSTIC TESTING WITH ULTRASOUND

Ultrasonography has widespread application in obstetrics, particularly in evaluation and management of the high-risk pregnancy. Because accurate dating of
pregnancy is critical in planning various evaluations and interventions, the earliest
application of ultrasound is its use in establishing correct gestational age.

Before ~6 weeks of menstrual age (time elapsed since the first day of the last
menstrual period), using standard transabdominal ultrasound equipment, the
presence or absence of a gestational sac and fetal pole can be demonstrated.
Between 6 and 14 weeks of gestation, the crown-rump length of the fetus can be
measured, yielding 95% confidence limits of ±4.7 days for one measurement. If
multiple measurements are taken, the accuracy is increased.

Between 12 and 24 weeks of gestation, dating usually is accomplished by measurement of the biparietal diameter of the fetal head or the fetal femur length. For
these measurements, the accuracy is considerably higher at 12–20 weeks (95%
confidence interval ±7–8 days) than at 20–24 weeks (95% confidence interval ±2
weeks). For this reason, if ultrasound-estimated gestational age is within such confidence intervals based on last menstrual period, it is customary not to change the
estimated date of delivery, assuming that the patient is relatively certain about her
last menstrual period and that her menses follow a fairly consistent pattern. After
28 weeks of gestation, ultrasound estimates of gestational age diminish in reliability because of the large week-to-week overlap in the measurements taken (American Academy of Pediatrics and the American College of Obstetricians and
Gynecologists 2007, American College of Obstetricians and Gynecologists 2009).

Once gestational age has been established, ultrasound also can be used to evaluate fetal anatomy. The presence of maternal diabetes carries with it a significant
increase in the likelihood of major congenital malformations, particularly when

## Table 8.1 Diagnostic Testing and Fetal Surveillance

| Test | Purpose | Optimal Gestational Age (weeks) | Comments |
|------|---------|-------------------------------|----------|
| Ultrasound | Establish gestational age (American Academy of Pediatrics and the American College of Obstetricians and Gynecologists 2007) | After 6 | Reliability: 6–9 weeks 6 days (±3 days) 10–13 weeks 6 days (±5 days) 14–20 weeks (±7 days) >20 weeks unreliable (±2–4 weeks) |
| | Screen for structural anomalies | Variable | Detects many anomalies but cannot guarantee normalcy |
| | Detect macrosomia and hydramnios | 26 weeks to term | Indications of fetal effects of maternal diabetes |
| α-fetoprotein (αFP) | Detect risk of open fetal defect | 15–20 | If elevated, possible open fetal defect (anencephaly, spina bifida, etc.) |
| Integrated screen, multiple markers, with or without nuchal translucency | Detect risk of certain aneuploidies | Part 1 at 10 weeks 3 days to 13 weeks; part 2 at 15–22 weeks 6 days | Detects risk of trisomy 21, 18, 13, and open fetal defects |
| Genetic testing on maternal or paternal blood sample | Detect carrier state for heritable diseases | Any | Look for a specific disease; currently available for Tay-Sachs, cystic fibrosis, sickle cell disease, thalassemia, and many others |
| Genetic amniocentesis | Test for chromosome abnormalities | >15 | Small risk of complications; diabetes does not cause chromosome abnormalities |
| Cell-free DNA testing of maternal blood | Test for trisomy 21 | >10 | Relatively new development; continues to evolve |
| Chorionic villus sampling | Test for chromosome abnormalities | >9 | Increased miscarriage rate |
| Fetal activity | Screen for fetal well-being | 28–40 | Simple, inexpensive |
| Nonstress testing | Screen for fetal well-being | 26–40 | False positive results in a sleeping, immature, or inactive fetus |

| Test | Purpose | Optimal Gestational Age (weeks) | Comments |
|---|---|---|---|
| Biophysical profile | Evaluate chronic and acute fetal problems using ultrasound | 26–40 | May be the most reliable |
| Amniocentesis | Test for fetal lung maturity | Preterm | Not often needed |
| Doppler velocimetry | Test for fetal umbilical blood flow in intrauterine growth restriction (IUGR) pregnancy | Third trimester | Best indicator of high risk of fetal demise in IUGR |

glucose control during organogenesis is not optimal. Although not all such malformations can be diagnosed with ultrasound, many can be found with a thorough fetal evaluation. The likelihood of finding abnormalities that are present increases if the a priori risk is known to be high, because the ultrasonographer is highly motivated in such cases to continue scanning until he or she is satisfied that no lesions can be found. Therefore, detailed ultrasound studies (also known as level II ultrasound or targeted ultrasound) should be carried out in diabetic pregnancies, especially in cases in which other risk factors are known to be present. Such risk factors include an elevated glycohemoglobin level at the time of first prenatal visit, high or low serum or amniotic fluid α-fetoprotein (αFP) (see the next section), or suggestive past history or family history of delivering a malformed infant. Although such scans can be performed in pregnancies without any of these risk factors, the sensitivity is likely to be reduced, and a negative result in no way guarantees fetal normalcy. Patients should be informed of these limitations before scanning.

## α-FETOPROTEIN TESTING

αFP, a fetal product that appears in both amniotic fluid and maternal circulation, often is present in increased concentration when an open fetal defect occurs (i.e., anencephaly, spinal defect, or ventral wall defect, such as omphalocele or gastroschisis). Its maternal concentration may be low in some cases of chromosomal aneuploidy (i.e., trisomy 21). αFP screening is best done at ~15–20 weeks of gestation because that is the time when it is most accurate.

Because maternal type 1 diabetes (T1D) is associated with an increased risk for the defects named thus far, among others, maternal serum αFP (MSαFP) screening generally is offered to such patients. The MSαFP level is expressed by the laboratory in multiples of the median (MOM) to standardize the results. Various centers recommend further testing at levels ≥2.0 or >2.5 MOM. Women with T1D have been reported to manifest lower MSαFP levels at a given gestational age compared with nondiabetic women. Some studies have linked this lowering of

MSαFP to poor metabolic control as manifested by elevated glycohemoglobin levels. Depending on the circumstances and patient preference, an elevated MSαFP may prompt either an amniocentesis (to measure amniotic fluid αFP) or a level II ultrasound examination.

Most centers offer "multiple-marker screening," in which measurements of the levels of substances other than αFP, such as human chorionic gonadatropin (hCG) and estriol, are made to improve the predictive value for chromosomal aneuploidies. Because maternal diabetes does not appear to increase the risk for such aneuploidies in the fetus, these multiple-marker tests should be considered equally appropriate for women with diabetes as for the general population. A further refinement in this area combines first-trimester screening (nuchal translucency measurement with or without serum markers, including PAPP-A, and β-hCG), which may be combined with multiple-marker screening in the second trimester (αFP, unconjugated estriol, inhibin-A, and β-hCG). When results of first trimester screening are combined with those of second-trimester screening to provide a single risk estimate the test is called an "Integrated Screen." When first trimester screening results are conveyed so that high-risk results can lead to further diagnostic testing while lower-risk results can be refined by second-trimester screening the test is called a "Sequential Screen." Further details are beyond the scope of this chapter, but readers are referred to an American College of Obstetricians and Gynecologists (ACOG 2007b) Practice Bulletin on the topic.

## GENETIC TESTING

Maternal diabetes does not increase the risk for genetically inherited diseases. Individuals with diabetes, however, like all prenatal patients, should be questioned about family history, including ethnic background, with an eye toward the identification of a high genetic risk. For example, patients of Ashkenazi Jewish or French Canadian descent are at increased risk of being carriers for Tay-Sachs disease, a uniformly fatal autosomal recessive disorder. In addition, maternal age is associated with an increased risk for chromosomal abnormalities. Mothers at the age of 35 years (diabetes does not change the relationship between maternal age and risk) have an ~1/180 chance of delivering a baby with a chromosomal abnormality; about half of these babies have Down's syndrome. The general population risk is ~1/1,000. Thus, any patients for whom age or family history suggest increased genetic risk should receive thorough genetic counseling.

Genetic amniocentesis, the most common method of genetic testing, is a procedure in which a needle is inserted transabdominally into the amniotic sac with ultrasound guidance to obtain amniotic fluid. Fetal cells separated from the amniotic fluid are grown in tissue culture for karyotyping (chromosome analysis) or other types of testing. This test is generally performed at 14–20 weeks of gestation, and the results of metaphase analysis of cultured cells may take from 1 to 2 weeks to return, depending on the tests desired and the laboratory facilities. Fluorescence in situ hybridization (FISH) analysis can provide more rapid results when specific chromosome number defects, such as those involving chromosome 21, 13, 18, or the sex chromosomes, are sought. False-negative and false-positive results may occur, however, so FISH results should be confirmed by karyotyping or the presence of such evidence as ultrasound markers for the particular defect or positive screening tests. Several different enzymatic defects also can be determined on fetal cells from amniotic fluid, but each requires the services of a specialized laboratory. Thus, it is necessary to know whether a particular couple is at risk for a particular genetic disease; there is no "screening" test on amniotic fluid that can detect all of the possible genetic diseases. When amniotic fluid is withdrawn for genetic testing, αFP usually is measured as well. There is a small but definite risk of an untoward event such as premature labor, rupture of the membranes, or fetal injury associated with amniocentesis, with a perinatal loss rate estimated at between 1/300 and 1/500; patients should be informed of these risks before the procedure. Further information on invasive prenatal testing may be found in an ACOG (2007a) Practice Bulletin.

Chorionic villus sampling (CVS), another method of obtaining tissue for genetic studies, involves taking a "biopsy" of the placenta, either via a catheter inserted into the uterus transvaginally or with a needle inserted transabdominally. CVS is available only in specialized centers. Its advantages include the facts that it can be accomplished earlier in pregnancy than amniocentesis, as early as 9 weeks, and that the results can be available in just a few days. For some couples, this decreases decision-making pressure, because first-trimester pregnancy terminations are safer and less traumatic to the mother. The primary disadvantage of CVS is that there is an increased pregnancy loss rate reported compared with amniocentesis, and a few case series have reported an excess of limb defects in the offspring, particularly with very early CVS and with inexperienced operators. Thus, couples interested in CVS should be referred to experienced centers and should undergo extensive counseling before the procedure (ACOG 2007a).

## FETAL SURVEILLANCE WITH ULTRASOUND

In addition to verifying gestational age and detecting major anatomic abnormalities in the fetus, ultrasound is a useful tool for the assessment of fetal growth and the estimation of fetal weight. Because the fetus of a mother with diabetes may be macrosomic (large for gestational age) or alternatively may be growth restricted (small for gestational age), particularly in the presence of maternal vascular disease or hypertension, it is useful to perform periodic measurements of fetal growth during the third trimester. Excessive amounts of amniotic fluid (polyhydramnios) also may complicate diabetic pregnancy and usually can be detected with ultrasound (Coomarasamy 2005, Langer 2005, Chauhan 2006, Nahum 2006, Farrell 2007, ACOG 2009).

## FETAL ACTIVITY DETERMINATIONS

Because a diminution of the frequency or intensity of fetal movement may be associated with fetal jeopardy, many centers instruct pregnant women (particularly those with high-risk pregnancies) to "track" fetal movement daily during the third trimester. Numerous systems are used, including the recording of the number of perceived fetal movements during a given period or the recording of the amount of time that elapses until a given number of movements are perceived. Whenever preset thresholds for fetal movement are not met, the patient is asked to come in for more sophisticated biophysical antepartum testing (see the next section).

## ANTEPARTUM FETAL MONITORING

Each time the uterus contracts during normal labor, the delivery of nutrients and oxygen to the fetus is diminished. Ordinarily, the fetus possesses sufficient redundancy in its reserves of these substances that the contraction has no ill effect. A fetus functioning "on the edge," however, with depleted placental reserves, may respond to each uterine contraction with a characteristic slowing of its heart rate, technically known as a "late deceleration" when viewed on an electronic fetal heart rate monitoring printout (Fig. 8.1). Such late decelerations, if repetitive, are considered to be nonreassuring, possibly reflecting fetal compromise during labor. Similar changes may be seen on fetal heart rate tracings of pregnant women who are not yet in spontaneous labor but who have had contractions artificially induced with an intravenous infusion of oxytocin. The oxytocin challenge test consists of the induction of at least three uterine contractions during a 10-min epoch. If all three contractions are followed by late decelerations of the fetal heart rate, the test is considered positive and indicative of a high likelihood of fetal compromise.

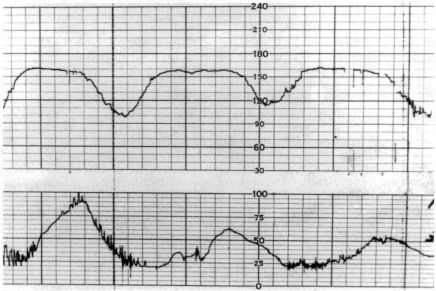

Top panel, fetal heart rate; bottom panel, uterine contractions. Note the fetal heart rate dip to 100 beats/min after contraction.

**Figure 8.1** Late Decelerations

In the course of the performance of thousands of records of fetal heart rate monitoring, it was noted that the healthy fetus usually demonstrated a transient increase in its heart rate after any vigorous fetal movement. The presence of two to three such accelerations of at least 15 beats/min, lasting at least 15 s, during a 20-min period is associated with a high likelihood of fetal well-being and is called a reactive nonstress test (NST) (Fig. 8.2). Because the NST requires only an electronic fetal monitor and not an intravenous infusion, it is easier to perform than the oxytocin challenge test and often is used as a primary test of fetal well-being. A reactive NST is a very strong indicator of fetal well-being, but a nonreactive NST may be seen in fetal sleep states, fetal immaturity, and other situations that are not necessarily adverse. Thus, a nonreactive NST usually is followed up by another fetoplacental function test, such as a biophysical profile.

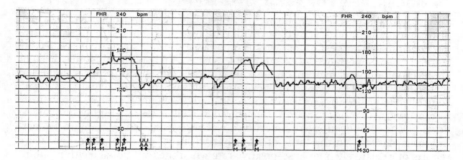

Note the rise in fetal heart rate (FHR) with each fetal movement (FM).

**Figure 8.2** Fetal Monitor Strip from Nonstress Test

The biophysical profile is thought to combine the evaluation of chronic and acute fetal problems. In this test, the NST is combined with an ultrasound evaluation of fetal movement, fetal tone (flexion of the extremities), amniotic fluid volume, and fetal breathing. Each category is assigned a score of 0 (bad) or 2 (good) points. A score of 8–10 is normal, 6 is equivocal and suggests possible fetal jeopardy or asphyxia, and 0–4 is abnormal and very strongly indicative of fetal compromise (ACOG 1999). The presence of oligohydramnios (amniotic fluid index [AFI] ≤5 cm or deepest vertical pocket ≤2 cm) is highly suggestive of chronic problems (or ruptured membranes) and requires further evaluation or delivery, depending on the gestational age and clinical circumstances (ACOG 1999). The "modified biophysical profile" consists of a NST plus the measurement of the AFI. If both are normal no further evaluation is needed at that time. If either or both are abnormal, further evaluation is recommended.

Different perinatal centers use different combinations of these antepartum tests in the evaluation of the diabetic pregnancy. There is no single approach on which there is universal agreement. Certain principles, however, are generally accepted. Most centers would not start any type of antepartum testing until a gestational age at which there is a possibility of fetal survival if delivery is accomplished. Thus, there is no point in doing any of these tests at 20 weeks of gestation.

Because all of these tests can yield false-positive results, they should not be performed if a particular patient has little risk of fetal problems; in such patients, the predictive accuracy of a positive test is poor. Thus, a particular center might defer antepartum testing until 35 weeks in a patient with well-controlled diabetes who has no vascular complications but might start at 28 weeks or even earlier in a poorly controlled patient who has nephropathy, hypertension, and a growth-restricted fetus. In addition, these tests should be performed in a center in which there is adequate day-to-day experience in the performance and interpretation of whatever approach is chosen. Finally, the interval of testing may vary from once per week to daily, depending on the circumstances of a particular patient.

## AMNIOCENTESIS FOR FETAL LUNG MATURITY DETERMINATION

Several early studies suggested that respiratory distress syndrome (RDS), which histologically manifests as hyaline membrane disease, occurs with increased frequency and at later gestational ages in infants of mothers with diabetes. Tissue culture experiments have linked this problem with fetal hyperinsulinemia, brought about by suboptimal maternal metabolic control. Subsequent reports suggested that the risk for RDS is closer to background rates when maternal diabetes is well controlled (Kjos 1990). The use of amniotic fluid biochemical analysis can identify fetuses at greatest risk for RDS if delivered as well as fetuses highly unlikely to develop this complication. Amniocentesis was at one time quite useful in evaluating lung maturity in the fetus of a mother with diabetes. Because there were reports of a relatively high false-positive rate when the traditional lecithin-sphingomyelin ratio was used, most centers test for the presence of phosphatidylglycerol as a highly reliable sign of lung maturity. A recent workshop sponsored by the National Institute of Child Health and Human Development and the Society for Maternal–Fetal Medicine (SMFM) recommended that amniocentesis be used only rarely in determining the timing of delivery in diabetic pregnancies (Spong 2011). The reasoning was that, if an indication for delivery is present, amniocentesis to assess fetal lung maturity would not be helpful. For women with preexisting diabetes or gestational diabetes whose glucose levels have been well controlled and who do not have other complications, delivery before 39 weeks was not recommended. Early delivery without amniocentesis was recommended when diabetes has been poorly controlled or vascular or other complications are present.

## TIMING AND MODE OF DELIVERY

At one time, it was fairly routine to deliver infants of mothers with diabetes at some arbitrary number of weeks before term to lessen the likelihood of unexplained fetal death in utero. Because of the need for early delivery when the uterine cervix was not yet "ripe" to facilitate induction of labor and because fetal macrosomia complicated a significant proportion of these pregnancies, cesarean section was the routine route of birth. The advent of antepartum testing, as described, allowed the identification of particular pregnancies at high risk for impending intrauterine fetal death, so that the less threatened fetuses could be allowed to continue nearer to term. Most important, modern approaches to metabolic normalization of the pregnant woman with diabetes have prevented fetal deterioration, so that early delivery is less likely to be necessary. Because pregnancies allowed to progress closer to term are more likely to result in vaginal delivery and because improved metabolic control has lowered, but not eliminated, the likelihood of fetal macrosomia, women with diabetes often can safely deliver vaginally. A retrospective study of all births to women with gestational diabetes in California delivering from 1997 through 2006 compared the infant mortality risk associated with delivery at a given gestational age to the risks of stillbirth plus infant mortality associated with waiting 1 more week to deliver (Rosenstein 2012). The risk of expectant management was lower than that of delivery at 36 weeks, although the difference was not statistically significant. At 37 and 38 weeks, the risks were similar. At 39 weeks, and at 40 weeks, the risks of expectant management of GDM for one more week were significantly higher than for delivery. For example, the mortality risk of delivery at 39 weeks was 8.7/10,000 versus 17.1/10,000 if the pregnancy was managed expectantly for 1 more week. The authors calculated that 1,311 patients with gestational diabetes would need to be delivered at 39 weeks to prevent one excess stillbirth.

## FETAL SURVEILLANCE DURING LABOR

Because preexisting diabetes represents a high-risk situation with an increased possibility of fetal compromise, the fetal condition should be evaluated continuously with an electronic fetal monitoring device once labor has been established.

## DIABETIC KETOACIDOSIS

An episode of diabetic ketoacidosis (DKA) carries a risk in excess of 50% for fetal death. Not only is maternal acidosis dangerous for the fetus, but so too is the usual dehydration that accompanies DKA. It is possible for DKA to occur in the third trimester of pregnancy with a potentially viable fetus in utero. Nonreassuring fetal heart rate tracings are very likely in such situations and can be frightening to the caregiver, because emergency cesarean section, a major surgical procedure, carries a high maternal mortality risk when performed on an individual in DKA. On the other hand, in most cases, the fetal tracing improves as the maternal DKA is corrected. For this reason, it is usually best to defer emergency cesarean section until the mother's condition has been normalized through aggressive treatment with intravenous fluids, insulin, and potassium. Once the mother's acid-base balance has been restored and ketosis has disappeared, the fetal heart rate tracing usually has normalized. If not, consideration then can be given to delivery for fetal indications (Montoro 2004).

## PRETERM LABOR

Pregnancy in a mother with diabetes, like other pregnancies, may be complicated by preterm labor. It is arguable as to whether this complication occurs more frequently when the mother has diabetes, and data are supportive of both points of view. When preterm labor occurs between 24 and 34 weeks, and delivery is anticipated within 7 days, corticosteroid administration is recommended to enhance fetal pulmonic maturity. Because the large doses of corticosteroid cause maternal hyperglycemia and may precipitate ketoacidosis, particularly in gravidas with T1D, frequent blood glucose determination should be carried out for ≥48 h. Insulin requirements can be expected to increase markedly, and intravenous insulin infusion may be necessary. Preterm labor often is treated acutely for up to 48 h with tocolytic agents to inhibit uterine contractions and allow time for the corticosteroids to take effect. Some of these, ritodrine and terbutaline, have β-adrenergic agonist properties that can cause maternal hyperglycemia, hypokalemia, pulmonary edema believed to be secondary to alveolar capillary leakage, electrocardiographic abnormalities, tachycardia, and other problems. Although such agents are not absolutely contraindicated in mothers with diabetes, they should be used with caution. Frequent monitoring of maternal circulating glucose levels (hourly for the first 4 h, every 2–4 h thereafter) and serum potassium, performance of an electrocardiogram before institution of these agents, and avoidance of excessive amounts of salt-containing intravenous fluids are all recommended. In mothers with T1D, it is customary to start a constant intravenous insulin infusion at a rate ranging from 2 to 7 units/h when β-mimetic tocolytics are used parenterally. A preferable option is to use a nonadrenergic tocolytic agent. Calcium channel blockers such as nifedipine commonly are used. Indomethacin, an effective tocolytic agent, has been associated with premature closure of the fetal ductus arteriosus and with oligohydramnios, particularly when used for >48 h. Intravenous magnesium sulfate also has been used in this situation and does not cause hyperglycemia or hypokalemia, but is not an effective tocolytic. It can cause respiratory depression when serum magnesium levels are too high, and its use has been associated with pulmonary edema in isolated cases. When delivery is anticipated before 32 weeks, however, intravenous magnesium sulfate is recommended during the hours before delivery for fetal neuroprotection to prevent cerebral palsy (ACOG/SMFM 2010). The mother with diabetes should not be denied tocolysis when it is indicated, but tocolytic agents should be used cautiously in such patients. A more detailed discussion of the treatment of preterm labor may be found in the ACOG (2012) Practice Bulletin on this topic.

## SELECTED READINGS

American Academy of Pediatrics and the American College of Obstetricians and Gynecologists: *Guidelines for Perinatal Care.* 6th ed. Washington, DC, AAP and ACOG, 2007, p. 100

American College of Obstetricians and Gynecologists: Management of preterm labor. ACOG Practice Bulletin No. 127. *Obstet Gynecol* 119:1308–1317, 2012

American College of Obstetricians and Gynecologists: Ultrasonography in pregnancy. ACOG Practice Bulletin No. 101. *Obstet Gynecol* 113:451–461, 2009 (reaffirmed 2011)

American College of Obstetricians and Gynecologists: Invasive prenatal testing for aneuploidy. ACOG Practice Bulletin No. 88. *Obstet Gynecol* 110:1450–1467, 2007 (reaffirmed 2009)

American College of Obstetricians and Gynecologists: Screening for fetal chromosomal abnormalities. ACOG Practice Bulletin No. 77. *Obstet Gynecol* 109:217–227, 2007 (reaffirmed 2011)

American College of Obstetricians and Gynecologists: Antepartum fetal surveillance. ACOG Practice Bulletin No. 9. *Int J Gynaecol Obstet* 68:175–185, 1999 (reaffirmed 2012)

American College of Obstetricians and Gynecologists/Society for Maternal–Fetal Medicine: Magnesium sulfate before anticipated preterm birth for neuroprotection. Committee Opinion No. 455. *Obstet Gynecol* 115:669–671, 2010

Spong CY, Mercer BM, D'Alton M, Kilpatrick S, Blackwell S, Saade G: Timing of indicated late-preterm and early-term birth. *Obstet Gynecol* 118:323–333, 2011

## REFERENCES

American Academy of Pediatrics and the American College of Obstetricians and Gynecologists: *Guidelines for Perinatal Care.* 6th ed. Washington, DC, AAP and ACOG, 2007, p. 100

American College of Obstetricians and Gynecologists: Management of preterm labor. ACOG Practice Bulletin No. 127. *Obstet Gynecol* 119:1308–1317, 2012

American College of Obstetricians and Gynecologists: Ultrasonography in pregnancy. ACOG Practice Bulletin No. 101. *Obstet Gynecol* 113:451–461, 2009 (reaffirmed 2011)

American College of Obstetricians and Gynecologists: Invasive prenatal testing for aneuploidy. ACOG Practice Bulletin No. 88. *Obstet Gynecol* 110:1450–1467, 2007 (reaffirmed 2009)

American College of Obstetricians and Gynecologists: Screening for fetal chromosomal abnormalities. ACOG Practice Bulletin No. 77. *Obstet Gynecol* 109:217–227, 2007 (reaffirmed 2011)

American College of Obstetricians and Gynecologists: Antepartum fetal surveillance. ACOG Practice Bulletin No. 9. *Int J Gynaecol Obstet* 68:175–185, 1999 (reaffirmed 2012)

American College of Obstetricians and Gynecologists/Society for Maternal–Fetal Medicine: Magnesium sulfate before anticipated preterm birth for neuroprotection. Committee Opinion No. 455. *Obstet Gynecol* 115:669–671, 2010

Chauhan SP, Parker D, Shields D, Sanderson M, Cole JH, Scardo JA: Sonographic estimate of birth weight among high-risk patients: feasibility and factors influencing accuracy. *Am J Obstet Gynecol* 195:601–606, 2006

Coomarasamy A, Connock M, Thornton J, Khan KS: Accuracy of ultrasound biometry in the prediction of macrosomia: a systematic quantitative review. *Br J Obstet Gynaecol* 112:1461–1466, 2005

Farrell T, Owen P, Kernaghan D, Ola B, Bruce C, Fraser R: Can ultrasound fetal biometry predict fetal hyperinsulinaemia at delivery in pregnancy complicated by maternal diabetes? *Eur J Obstet Gyncol Reprod Biol* 131:146–150, 2007

Kjos SL, Walther FJ, Montoro M, et al.: Prevalence and etiology of respiratory distress syndrome in infants of diabetic mothers: predictive value of fetal lung maturation tests. *Am J Obstet Gynecol* 163:898–903, 1990

Langer O: Ultrasound biometry evolves in the management of diabetes in pregnancy. *Ultrasound Obstet Gynecol* 26:585–595, 2005

Montoro MM: Diabetic ketoacidosis in pregnancy. In *Diabetes in Women: Adolescence, Pregnancy, and Menopause*. Reece EA, Coustan DR, Gabbe SG, Eds. Philadelphia, PA, Lippincott Williams & Wilkins, 2004, p. 345–350

Nahum GG, Stanislaw H: Accurate prediction of fetal macrosomia using combination methods. *Am J Obstet Gynecol* 195:879–880, 2006

Rosenstein MG, Cheng YW, Snowden JM, et al.: The risk of stillbirth and infant death stratified by gestational age in women with gestational diabetes. *Am J Obstet Gynecol* 206:309.e1–e7, 2012

Spong CY, Mercer BM, D'Alton M, Kilpatrick S, Blackwell S, Saade G: Timing of indicated late-preterm and early-term birth. *Obstet Gynecol* 118:323–333, 2011

# Gestational Diabetes Mellitus

# Highlights
## Gestational Diabetes Mellitus

■ The definition of gestational diabetes mellitus (GDM) is glucose intolerance of variable severity, with onset or first recognition during the current pregnancy. This definition applies regardless of the need for insulin or whether the diabetes disappears after the pregnancy.

■ Any woman at high risk of diabetes (marked obesity, personal history of GDM, glycosuria, or a strong family history of diabetes) should be tested for diabetes using standard diagnostic criteria as soon as possible after confirmation of pregnancy.

■ All women who have not already been diagnosed with preexisting diabetes or gestational diabetes should undergo a 75-g, 2-h oral glucose tolerance test at 24–28 weeks gestation. Any one or more elevated value (fasting ≥92 mg/dl [5.1 mmol/l]; 1-h ≥180 mg/dl [10.0 mmol/l]; 2-h ≥153 mg/dl [8.5 mmol/l]) makes the diagnosis of gestational diabetes.

■ The mainstay of therapy is the dietary prescription. The goal of medical nutrition therapy (MNT) is to keep the peak postprandial glucose response in the normal range.

■ Glucose monitoring is paramount in the woman with gestational diabetes. Criteria for beginning insulin are based on the fasting and postprandial responses to the prescribed meal plan.

■ When indicated by fasting or postprandial glucose levels, therapy with insulin is prescribed to reestablish normoglycemia.

■ Exercise programs are considered safe as an adjunct therapy for GDM.

■ Timing and mode of delivery are determined not only by the classic obstetric indications but also by the glycemic control of the mother.

■ Postpartum, insulin requirements will disappear, and in most women, the diabetes will disappear. A glucose tolerance test 6–8 weeks postpartum should be performed to ensure that the woman is not left with prediabetes or type 2 diabetes (T2D).

■ A prevention program should be started immediately postpartum to keep the woman lean and fit, which markedly decreases the chances that she will develop T2D as she ages.

# Gestational Diabetes Mellitus

Gestational diabetes mellitus (GDM) is defined as carbohydrate intolerance of variable severity with onset or first recognition during pregnancy. The definition applies regardless of whether insulin is used for treatment or the condition persists after pregnancy (Metzger 1991). The broad definition of GDM allows for a potentially heterogeneous group of patients. It is possible that some women with GDM may have had unrecognized diabetes, either type 1 diabetes (T1D) or type 2 diabetes (T2D), antedating pregnancy (Omori 2005). Because GDM typically is a disorder of late gestation, this possibility is particularly great if hyperglycemia is noted during the first trimester. Insulin resistance is a characteristic of all pregnancies, presumably based on fetal–placental hormone production and release. Although most pregnant women increase insulin production to maintain euglycemia in response to this phenomenon, some are unable to sufficiently augment their insulin response, or are more insulin resistant than average, and develop hyperglycemia that is labeled gestational diabetes.

Maternal hyperglycemia and a surfeit of other metabolic fuels (i.e., plasma lipids and amino acids) increase the risk of macrosomia, birth trauma, and neonatal hypoglycemia. Furthermore, the effects of GDM appear to go well beyond the perinatal period to include long-range implications for future diabetes, obesity, and abnormal neurobehavioral development (Silverman 1991).

## DIAGNOSIS

The diagnostic criteria for gestational diabetes differ widely around the globe and are a topic of current debate. In various countries, the glucose tolerance test utilizes a 50-g, 75-g, or 100-g challenge; it may last for 2 h or 3 h; the diagnosis may require one elevated value or two elevated values. The thresholds may be based on the likelihood of subsequent diabetes in the mother (O'Sullivan 1964) or simply utilize the same cutoffs as in nonpregnant individuals (World Health Organization 2012). In response to the need for globally accepted, pregnancy outcome–based, standardized criteria for diagnosing gestational diabetes, the Hyperglycemia and Adverse Pregnancy Outcome (HAPO) study reported on the results of blinded 75-g, 2-h oral glucose tolerance tests (OGTTs) administered to >23,000 pregnant women around the world (HAPO Study Cooperative Research Group 2008). Each of the three OGTT plasma glucose values (fasting, 1-h, and 2-h) was related to each of the primary outcomes (fetal macrosomia, fetal hyperinsulinemia, primary cesarean section, and neonatal hypoglycemia) in a linear and significant manner. Similar relationships were found with secondary outcomes such as pre-eclampsia, shoulder dystocia, and birth injury. Because there was no obvious inflection point in these relationships, recommendations for diagnostic criteria were made by a panel of experts from various countries, assembled by the International Association of Diabetes in Pregnancy Study Groups (Metzger 2010). The criteria were based on the glucose values at each of the three time points, which were associated with odds ratios of 1.75 for macrosomia, fetal hyperinsulinemia, and neonatal body fat above the 90th percentile. On the basis of similar levels of risk for adverse outcomes associated with each of the three OGTT values, a single elevated value was sufficient to make the diagnosis of gestational diabetes. In 2011 the American Diabetes Association (ADA) recommended these new OGTT criteria in the "Standards of Medical Care in Diabetes—2011" (ADA 2011), and the information in this chapter is based on these recommendations. Other professional organizations have not yet adopted these criteria, however, and there are likely regional and local differences in how the diagnosis of gestational diabetes is approached.

The newly recommended criteria are expected to increase the prevalence of gestational diabetes in the U.S. to the range of 15–25% of pregnant women (Sacks 2012). It is not clear whether the same intensity of monitoring and treatment will be necessary for these newly diagnosed, milder forms of gestational diabetes.

Medical care for women with GDM begins with detection. The ADA recommends that any pregnant women with risk factors for diabetes (marked obesity, personal history of GDM, glycosuria, or a strong family history of diabetes) be tested for diabetes at the first prenatal visit, using standard diagnostic criteria (ADA 2013). For women who are not found to have diabetes in early pregnancy, and for all other pregnant women, it is recommended they be tested for GDM at 24–28 weeks of gestation, using a 75-g, 2-h OGTT, and the diagnostic cut points listed in Table 9.1. The test is performed in the morning after an overnight fast of at least 8 h but not >14 h. Once the diagnosis has been established, patients should be counseled about diet, exercise, self-monitoring of blood glucose (SMBG), obstetric care, and in some cases, administration of insulin.

---

## EPIDEMIOLOGY

The prevalence of GDM varies markedly in different parts of the world and among racial and ethnic groups within the same country, even when the same diagnostic criteria are utilized. Among the >23,000 participants in the HAPO study, from 15 centers in 9 different countries around the world, GDM would have been diagnosed in 9–25% of pregnant women (Sacks 2012).

Although most women with GDM return to normal glucose tolerance postpartum, the disorder is clearly associated with an increased risk of subsequent overt diabetes. Women in whom GDM was diagnosed should be tested for persistent diabetes at 6–12 weeks postpartum, using a test other than A1C. They should be educated regarding the symptoms of overt diabetes and should have lifelong screening for the development of diabetes or prediabetes at least every 3 years.

## Table 9.1 Diagnosis of Preexisting Diabetes in Pregnancy and Gestational Diabetes

- At the first prenatal visit, women at risk for diabetes should be tested using one of the standard diagnostic criteria:
  - Fasting plasma glucose ≥126 mg/dl, or
  - A1C ≥6.5%, or
  - 2-h plasma glucose ≥200 mg/dl on a 75-gram OGTT, or
  - Random plasma glucose ≥200 mg/dl in a patient with classic symptoms of hyperglyce-mia
  - A positive test should be confirmed by repeat testing unless it is unequivocal.
  - Women whose initial test is not diagnostic of diabetes, but whose fasting plasma glu-cose is ≥92 mg/dl but <126 mg/dl may be diagnosed with gestational diabetes.
- Pregnant women not known to have diabetes or gestational diabetes should be tested at 24–28 weeks' gestation, using a 75-g, 2-h OGTT. Gestational diabetes is diagnosed if at least one of the following thresholds is met or exceeded:
  - Fasting plasma glucose ≥92 mg/dl
  - 1-h plasma glucose ≥180 mg/dl
  - 2-h plasma glucose ≥153 mg/dl

## NUTRITIONAL MANAGEMENT

Nutritional counseling is the cornerstone of the management of all women with GDM and is based on the standard nutritional recommendations for pregnant women. The principles are similar to those outlined in chapter 6 for pregnant women with preexisting diabetes. All women with GDM should receive nutritional counseling by a registered dietitian when possible. In the management of GDM, medical nutrition therapy (MNT), provided by a registered dietitian, results in decreased hospital admissions and insulin use, improves the likelihood of normal fetal and placental growth, and reduces the risk of perinatal complications, especially when diagnosed and treated early. Initial interventions should occur as soon as possible after diagnosis (within 1 week) and should include follow-up visits (Reader 2006, Academy of Nutrition and Dietetics 2008). Individualization of MNT depending on maternal weight and height is recommended (ADA 2004). The nutrition plan is effective if it achieves the following:

- Provides the necessary nutrients for maternal–fetal health
- Results in normoglycemia
- Prevents ketosis
- Results in appropriate weight gain

### GOALS

Although normoglycemia is the accepted goal of managing gestational diabetes, the means to that end remain controversial. Dietary management has been used in the treatment of pregnancies complicated by diabetes since the 19th century. Since 1898, diets prescribed for individuals with diabetes have ranged from extremely high fat (85% of calories) to undernutrition and fasting. From the early insulin years (1922–1940) to the present, the carbohydrate content of the diabetic diet has steadily risen from 35% of calories to the previously recommended level of 55–60% of calories (Peterson 1991). The ADA now recommends individualizing the carbohydrate content of the diet to achieve normoglycemia.

Specifically, the ADA recommends that women with GDM receive nutritional recommendations on the basis of an individual nutritional assessment. Dietitians base their guidelines for nutritional management on a combination of nutrient requirements in pregnancy combined with dietary management of diabetes and SMBG.

The goals of MNT in GDM are as follows:

■ Achieve and maintain normoglycemia, defined as fasting plasma glucose ≤95 mg/dl (≤5.3 mmol/l), 1-h postprandial plasma glucose ≤140 mg/dl (≤7.8 mmol/l), and 2-h postprandial plasma glucose ≤120 mg/dl (≤6.7 mmol/l).

■ Provide a nutritionally adequate diet for pregnancy. A nutritionally adequate diet contains all the essential nutrients required for fetal development and maintenance of maternal health. It also provides sufficient calories for the woman to achieve an appropriate weight gain and for her to avoid ketonuria.

## FACTORS AFFECTING BLOOD GLUCOSE LEVELS

Tight control of blood glucose levels is necessary during pregnancy because the fetus can be affected adversely by maternal hyperglycemia. The following factors affect blood glucose levels:

■ Stress (physical stress in the form of trauma, inflammation, infection, or hormonal imbalance due to growth and development, menstrual cycle, or pregnancy; exogenously administered steroids; and psychological stress)
■ Time of day
■ Exercise
■ Amount of carbohydrate eaten

Stress, both psychological and physical, increases blood glucose levels via contrainsulin hormones, including during pregnancy. Pregnancy increases the normal morning glucose intolerance caused by high levels of cortisol, progesterone, and human placental lactogen. For this reason, hyperglycemia after breakfast commonly occurs in GDM unless carbohydrate is restricted. Greater percentages of carbohydrate can be tolerated later in the day.

The time of day also affects blood glucose levels because of the diurnal variation of contrainsulin hormones. Exercise decreases blood glucose levels by increasing the uptake of glucose into the cells without extra insulin.

The amount of carbohydrate consumed in a meal or snack is highly correlated with the effect on blood glucose (Peterson 1991, Major 1998). The greater the percentage of carbohydrate in the meal, the higher the resultant blood glucose level. Women diagnosed with GDM often are motivated to maintain normal blood glucose with nutrition therapy. Carbohydrate intake has a direct effect on postprandial glucose levels. Although there is no ideal amount of carbohydrate recommended, controlling the carbohydrate amount and type can affect blood glucose levels. The routine use of SMBG enables women with GDM to include foods based on their individual postprandial glucose response, nutrient adequacy, and personal preference. Weight loss is not recommended (National Research Council 2009), and minimum carbohydrate recommendations are 175 g/day (Institute of Medicine, Food and Nutrition Board 2006; Reader 2007).

## DIETARY GUIDELINES

It is helpful to provide women with basic dietary guidelines ("dos and don'ts") *1)* to promote normoglycemia and avoid excessive weight gain and *2)* to develop an individual meal plan with the patient. The rationale for each recommendation is briefly described as follows:

- **Avoid concentrated sweets.**
  *Rationale*: These foods cause hyperglycemia in women with GDM; they are usually high in calories and low in nutrients. Emphasize fresh foods.
- **Avoid highly processed foods.**
  *Rationale*: Eating highly processed foods usually results in a more rapid rise in blood glucose than fresh or less processed foods. These foods are often high in fat, contributing to excessive weight gain.
- **Eat small meals.**
  *Rationale*: Consuming small frequent meals helps women avoid postprandial hyperglycemia and preprandial starvation ketosis. A consistent meal pattern is important: three meals and three snacks usually are recommended. Snacks prevent women from becoming overly hungry and overeating at the next meal. Protein foods are encouraged because they are digested and absorbed more slowly than carbohydrates, yielding a lower glycemic response. The fat in protein foods contributes to a greater satiety value than carbohydrate-rich foods, preventing excessive hunger. The small frequent meal pattern also helps to alleviate nausea and heartburn, two common discomforts of pregnancy.
- **Eat a small breakfast.**
  *Rationale*: A small breakfast, low in carbohydrate (<10%), is needed because morning blood glucose levels are likely to be high in patients with GDM. Fruits and juices should be avoided; milk should be limited (or omitted if postprandial hyperglycemia results). Highly processed breakfast cereals should be excluded.
- **Free foods (eat as desired)**: celery, lettuce, broccoli, cauliflower, nopales cactus, asparagus, tomatoes, etc.
  *Rationale:* These foods provide <20 kcal/serving, are very low in carbohydrate, and may be eaten when patients are hungry. These foods can be prepared as soups or eaten raw as salads.

## INDIVIDUALIZED MEAL PLANNING

*Composition of the diet.* ADA recommends that the dietary prescription be based on nutritional assessment and treatment goals. There is no standard "ADA diet." The recommended composition of the diet for women with GDM is to minimize the carbohydrate content of the meal plan and thus minimize the postprandial glucose excursions.

Within this prescription, complex carbohydrates, monounsaturated and poly-unsaturated fats, and foods high in fiber are encouraged. With this attention to carbohydrate intake, normoglycemia is maintained in 75–80% of women with gestational diabetes, whereas a higher carbohydrate intake results in more fre-quent episodes of hyperglycemia, with more women requiring insulin.

*Developing the meal plan.* Distribution of calories has been a source of contro-versy. Many programs recommend three meals and three snacks, regardless of whether the patient is taking insulin. Others feel that an overweight patient with GDM achieves better glucose control by simply consuming three meals and a bed-time snack (to prevent nocturnal ketone production).

Snacks can be advantageous. Protein-containing snacks between meals pre-vent extreme hunger at the next meal, and smaller meals and snacks every few hours are easier for pregnant women to digest.

The meal pattern is developed on an individual basis, based on the nutritional assessment of the patient. The diet must be consistent with the patient's lifestyle, food preferences, and cultural habits. A qualified educator, preferably a registered dietitian, should teach the patient, emphasizing appropriate portion sizes. Next, the educator should determine the appropriate calorie level and the amount of carbohydrate, protein, and fat for the individual. The educator then should record the number of servings from each food group to include in the daily diet. With the patient, the educator needs to develop a sample menu. To verify that the patient understands the meal plan, the patient should be asked to plan another sample menu, using a resource such as *Choose Your Foods: Plan Your Meals* or *Choose Your Foods: Exchange Lists for Meal Planning*.

## CONTROVERSY: CALORIE RESTRICTION FOR OBESE PATIENTS

In 2009 the Institute of Medicine (IOM) revised its recommendations for weight gain during pregnancy (National Research Council 2009). Women of normal prepregnancy weight (BMI 18.5–24.9) are advised to gain 25–35 lb; those who are overweight (BMI 25–29.9) are advised to gain 15–25 lb; obese individuals are advised to gain 11–20 lb. This was the first time that the IOM included upper limits for weight gain in pregnancy. A recent area of interest is the use of hypocaloric diets for obese women with GDM. One study indicated that restricting calories by 30–33% results in reduced hyperglycemia, reduced plasma triglycerides, and no increase in ketonuria, whereas a 50% reduction in caloric intake was associated with ketonuria (Knopp 1991). Other studies showed that calorie restriction (1,200–1,800 calories/day) normalized birth weights in babies of mothers with GDM with no increase in perinatal morbidity, although urinary ketones were not measured (Dornhorst 1991). Also, fewer women required insulin. One explanation for these results is that the women experienced an improvement in insulin sensitivity secondary to calorie restriction. The women in this study gained only 1.7 ± 1.6 kg (3.7 ± 3.5 lb) during the third trimester. Another potential advantage of calorie restriction is less postpartum obesity. The calorie-restricted approach might decrease the concentration of all maternal fuels reaching the fetal circulation (amino acids, plasma triglyceride fatty acids, and glucose), thereby reducing macrosomia. Levels of free fatty acids and ketones may increase, however, so further research is needed to determine whether calorie restriction might adversely affect the future health of the infant. In an observational study of 223 pregnant women (preexisting diabetes 40%; GDM 44%; normal glucose metabolism 16%), third-trimester β-hydroxybutyrate levels, which did not differ among the three groups, correlated inversely with mental development index scores in the offspring at 2 years of age and with Stanford-Binet scores at 3–5 years of age (Rizzo 1991). Such data give pause to efforts to impose caloric restriction in pregnancy severe enough to cause elevated ketone levels.

Currently, there is no scientifically validated method to estimate energy requirements in overweight and obese women. In clinical practice and some research protocols, the caloric prescription used for obese women is 25 kcal/kg and for normal-weight women is 35 kcal/kg based on prepregnancy weight (Diabetes Care and Education Practice Group 2007). Some practitioners use the Harris Benedict equation (with adjustments), and some use in-depth nutrition assessment, weight history, and clinical judgment. No matter the method used, the monitoring of nutrient adequacy, weight-gain patterns, and blood glucose levels should be ongoing and adjusted based on outcome measures.

## RECORDKEEPING AND FOLLOW-UP

The patient should be taught to keep food and blood glucose records, recording the time of the meal or snack and the amount and kinds of foods and beverages consumed. Checking blood glucose four times a day is recommended:

- Fasting (after rising)
- 1 or 2 h after breakfast
- 1 or 2 h after lunch
- 1 or 2 h after dinner

Although daily SMBG has been standard for individuals with gestational diabetes, it may be reasonable to utilize less frequent monitoring in patients with milder forms of this condition under the new diagnostic guidelines. A retrospective review of daily SMBG records demonstrated that, after a week of daily SMBG, every other day or every third day testing would not lead to significant delays in the initiation of insulin therapy in 120 individuals with mild gestational diabetes (fasting plasma glucose <95 mg/dl) (Mendez-Figueroa 2013).

The diet prescription should be validated with SMBG: the diet only "fits" if little or no postprandial hyperglycemia results (1-h postprandial blood glucose <140 mg/dl or 2-h values <120 mg/dl). The food records also help the registered dietitian to know whether the patient understands the diet. The records should be evaluated at every visit to provide vital feedback to the patient. The records are important for the following reasons:

- Individual food sensitivities can be pinpointed (e.g., foods that yield a high glycemic response).
- They allow the registered dietitian to evaluate the patient's understanding of the meal plan and to provide appropriate continuing education.
- Perhaps most important, they help the patient learn to make decisions about what and how much to eat, putting her in control.

Prenatal vitamin supplements often are used in pregnancy, because it is difficult to assess the adequacy of micronutrient intake. Iron is recommended as an additional nutritional supplement in women with iron deficiency anemia.

## POSTPARTUM

Women with GDM have a 40–60% chance of developing T2D as they age (Metzger 1991). When women with prediabetes, who had previous gestational diabetes, were randomized to metformin treatment, lifestyle intervention, or placebo, the annual incidence of conversion to diabetes was 15% in the placebo group, but was cut in half by either of the two treatments (Ratner 2008). The number needed to treat with lifestyle intervention to prevent one case of diabetes over 3 years was 5. With an appropriate weight-loss and fitness program, these women can improve their health and lower their risk of developing diabetes.

Breast-feeding should be encouraged in women with GDM. Breast-feeding has numerous physiological and emotional advantages over formula feeding. Although not all women lose weight while breast-feeding, it is normal for weight loss to occur because of a greater energy expenditure during lactation.

## EXERCISE AS A TREATMENT MODALITY

GDM is considered to be in part a disorder of glucose utilization, although it has been shown that this disorder is a heterogeneous entity (Freinkel 1985). A treatment modality that overcomes the peripheral resistance to insulin, such as exercise, should reduce the need for insulin administration. Cardiovascular conditioning exercise facilitates glucose utilization among other things by increasing insulin binding to and affinity for its receptor and receptor number (Pederson 1980).

Exercise during pregnancy is widely accepted (American College of Obstetricians and Gynecologists [ACOG] 2002). The safest form of exercise is that which does not cause fetal distress, low infant birth weight, uterine contractions, or maternal hypertension (blood pressure >140/90 mmHg) (Pomerance 1974, Artal 1984, Collings 1985, Jovanovic 1985, Carpenter 1988). Women may be taught to palpate their own uterus during exercise and stop the exercise if they detect a contraction. In addition to proper frequency, intensity, duration, and modality of exercise, self-monitoring of uterine activity may be a means of surveillance that allows the safe prescription of exercise during the third trimester.

Upper-body cardiovascular training has resulted in lower levels of glycemia than in women treated by diet only (Jovanovic-Peterson 1989, Durak 1990). The effects of exercise on glucose metabolism can become apparent after 4 weeks of training and affect both hepatic glucose output (reflected by fasting glucose levels) and glucose utilization (reflected by glucose values after a 50-g oral glucose challenge) (Jovanovic-Peterson 1989). Evidence also suggests that exercise may help to prevent gestational diabetes, particularly in obese women (Dye 1997). Pregnant women should not engage in contact sports such as hockey, football, or soccer, where injury is likely, or in activities with a high potential for falling, such as downhill skiing or gymnastics.

## METABOLIC MANAGEMENT DURING PREGNANCY

An Australian randomized controlled trial RCT (Crowther 2005) demonstrated that identifying and treating mild GDM (diagnosed when the 2-h value after a 75-g oral glucose load was 140–198 mg/dl [7.8–11.0 mmol/l] and mean fasting plasma glucose was 86 ± 13 mg/dl [4.8 ± 0.7 mmol/l]) significantly reduced the likelihood of a composite of serious neonatal morbidities compared with routine prenatal care. Macrosomia, preeclampsia, and other adverse outcomes were significantly less frequent as well. Treatment included individualized MNT, daily SMBG, and insulin, which was needed in 20% of those randomized to diagnosis and treatment. Another RCT conducted by the National Institute of Child Health and Human Development (NICHD) Maternal-Fetal Medicine (MFM) Units Network compared patients with mild GDM using the previous diagnostic criteria of Carpenter and Coustan, but normal fasting plasma glucose (<95 mg/dl), who were diagnosed and treated, to those whose GDM was not diagnosed (Landon 2009). Those who were diagnosed and treated, of whom 8% required insulin, were significantly less likely to experience preeclampsia, cesarean section, or shoulder dystocia, or to have macrosomic offspring. These studies constitute level 1 evidence that the diagnosis and treatment, even of mild forms of gestational diabetes, can significantly improve pregnancy outcomes.

### INTENSIFIED METABOLIC THERAPY

To determine whether dietary management is effective in maintaining euglycemia, blood glucose concentration must be monitored regularly. The use of insulin is widely recommended when appropriate MNT does not consistently maintain normal fasting plasma glucose ≤95 mg/dl (≤5.3 mmol/l), 1-h postprandial glucose <140 mg/dl (7.8 mmol/l), or 2-h postprandial plasma glucose ≤120 mg/dl (≤6.7 mmol/l). An isolated glucose level often can be attributed to a temporary dietary indiscretion. More frequent measurements exceeding the recommended goals, however, should prompt either the reassessment of glycemia within the next few days or the institution of insulin therapy. One approach is to start insulin when one-third or more of a week's values (fasting and or after any particular mealtime) exceed goals.

To safely initiate insulin therapy, qualified educators teach the basic timing and action of insulin; proper injection technique; dietary adjustments; and recognition, avoidance, and treatment of hypoglycemia. No data demonstrate superiority of a particular insulin regimen in GDM. It is recommended that insulin administration be individualized to achieve the glycemic goals stated previously.

*Human insulin* is the least immunogenic of the commercially available preparations, but the three rapid-acting insulin analogs (lispro, aspart, and glulisine) are comparable in immunogenicity to human regular insulin. Insulin preparations of low antigenicity will minimize the transplacental transport of insulin antibodies. Of the three rapid- and short-acting insulin analogs, only lispro and aspart have been investigated in pregnancy, with acceptable safety profiles, minimal transfer across the placenta, and no evidence of teratogenesis. These two insulin analogs both improve postprandial excursions compared with human regular insulin and are associated with lower risk of delayed postprandial hypoglycemia. An RCT has evaluated the use of the long-acting insulin analog detemir in pregnancy and it is Food and Drug Administration (FDA) Category B. Insulin glargine is FDA Category C in pregnancy, although it is unlikely to cross the placenta (Pollex 2010). Human neutral protamine Hagedorn (NPH) insulin most often is used as part of a multiple injection regimen for intermediate-acting insulin effect in GDM.

Regarding oral *antihyperglycemic agents*, of the sulfonylurea drugs, glyburide (glibenclamide) originally was believed to have minimal (4%) transfer across the human placenta (Elliott 1991) and has not been associated with excess neonatal hypoglycemia in the few studies available. A subsequent study, however, demonstrated that cord blood levels of glyburide were 70% of simultaneous maternal levels (Hebert 2009). Although there is no evidence, to date, of adverse outcomes in the newborn associated with maternal glyburide use, long-term studies are not available, necessitating appropriate patient counseling when this medication is prescribed during pregnancy. Glyburide must be balanced carefully with meals and snacks to prevent maternal hypoglycemia (as with insulin therapy). There is some evidence that glyburide may be less successful in obese patients or patients with marked hyperglycemia earlier in pregnancy. As with MNT/physical activity and insulin regimens, SMBG and fetal measurements of abdominal circumference (AC) or other parameters of fetal size need to be followed closely in women using glyburide. More research is needed to determine *1*) if maternal and neonatal outcomes with glyburide are equivalent to those obtained with insulin therapy; *2*) if there are glyburide effects on the potential postpartum progression of the woman with GDM toward glucose intolerance or diabetes, or on the possibility of GDM recurrence; and *3*) whether there are glyburide effects on the well-being of offspring in the medium and long term.

Metformin does cross the placenta, with cord levels measured at approximately twice maternal levels (Vanky 2005). A randomized trial comparing metformin to insulin in women with gestational diabetes requiring treatment demonstrated similar outcomes in both groups (Rowan 2008). Although patients randomized to metformin expressed a preference for this mode of therapy in future pregnancies, almost half required the addition of insulin to meet glucose targets. Metformin did not prevent GDM in a randomized trial (Vanky 2010).

Acarbose, an α-glucosidase inhibitor, is poorly absorbed from the gastrointestinal tract, and two preliminary studies have suggested efficacy in reducing postprandial glucose excursions in GDM, but with the expected frequency of abdominal cramping (Zárate 2000, de Veciana 2002). Because a small proportion of this drug may be absorbed systemically, further study should evaluate potential transplacental passage. Use of thiazolidinediones, glinides, and glucagon-like peptide (GLP)-1 during pregnancy is considered experimental. No controlled data are available in pregnancy, and one study reported that rosiglitazone crossed the human placenta at 10–12 weeks of gestation, with fetal tissue levels measured at about half of maternal serum levels (Chan 2005). With regard to GLP-1 agonists, ex vivo human placental perfusion studies detected minimal levels on the fetal side (fetal-to-maternal ratio 0.017) (Hiles 2003).

## GOALS AND SURVEILLANCE

Recommended goals for glucose control are similar to those outlined in chapter 4 for pregnancy in women with preexisting diabetes (Metzger 2007):

- Fasting glucose <96 mg/dl
- 1-h glucose <140 mg/dl
- 2-h glucose <120 mg/dl

There are no data from controlled trials of lower versus higher targets or 1-h versus 2-h postprandial testing to identify ideal goals for the prevention of fetal risks. Evidence from observational studies suggests that when *mean* capillary glucose levels in GDM are low (<87 mg/dl [<4.8 mmol/l]), there is an increased likelihood of infants who are small for gestational age (Langer 1994). An RCT comparing preprandial and postprandial glucose testing in GDM demonstrated that basing therapeutic decisions on postprandial goals (1-hr <140 mg/dl) reduced adverse outcomes compared with the use of preprandial goals (60–105 mg/dl) (de Veciana 1995). Daily SMBG using meters with memory capability appears to be superior to less frequent monitoring in the clinic for detection of glucose concentrations that may warrant intensification of therapy beyond individualized MNT. Many providers decrease the frequency of SMBG when MNT is successful in achieving goals for metabolic control; available data do not address such issues as the duration of good control sufficient to reduce the frequency of SMBG or the appropriate frequency of testing in women with GDM who are well controlled on MNT. As noted, with the anticipated increase in the prevalence of gestational diabetes as new diagnostic criteria are put into common use, patients with milder forms of this disorder may be able to monitor their glucose less frequently. New technologies for glucose surveillance should enable future research to determine optimal goals for metabolic control. Although not recommended in pregnancy, if alternative site testing is used, consideration should be given to the lag time for changes in postprandial glucose when compared with fingerstick capillary glucose testing. Validation of the accuracy of patients' monitoring techniques is also essential.

Assessing the fetal response to maternal GDM by ultrasound measurement of fetal AC starting in the second and early third trimesters and repeated every 3–6 weeks can provide useful information (in combination with maternal SMBG levels) to guide management decisions (Parretti 2001). Tighter glycemic control targets may be selected when size of the fetal abdomen is excessive, or pharmacological therapy can be added or intensified if a large AC is detected despite seemingly good glycemic control (Buchanan 1998, Kjos 2001). For this approach to be effective in clinical practice, attention should be given to the accuracy of the measurements of fetal size and maternal glucose. More prospective studies are needed to assess the cost-effectiveness of this approach compared with SMBG continued throughout pregnancy. Further study should address the addition of other measures of fetal size (subcutaneous fat and head circumference–to-AC ratio) to the assessment of the fetal response to maternal management (Buchanan 1998, Kjos 2001).

Urine ketone testing has been recommended in GDM patients with severe hyperglycemia, weight loss during treatment, or other concerns of possible "starvation ketosis." Fingerstick blood ketone testing is available and is more representative of laboratory measurements of β-hydroxybutyrate. The effectiveness of ketone monitoring (either urine or blood) in improving fetal outcome has not been tested, however. Insufficient data are available to determine whether measurement of glycosylated hemoglobin or other circulating proteins are of value in the routine management of GDM. An observational study of women with severe gestational diabetes (A1C >7.0% [estimated average glucose 155 mg/dl], average A1C 8.8% [estimated average glucose 206 mg/dl] at time of GDM diagnosis) found an average fall in A1C of 0.47% per week after diet and insulin therapy were begun (Jovanovic 2010). It is highly likely that all or most of these patients had preexisting diabetes; the utility of frequent A1C measurement in patients with gestational diabetes remains uncertain.

Most women with GDM will not require insulin during labor because the exercise of labor uses glucose substrate. Nevertheless, it is important to continue measuring blood glucose to detect the patients who do require insulin. When induction of labor is planned, insulin and breakfast should be omitted in the morning and intravenous fluids begun. Typically, fluids consist of 5% dextrose in half-normal saline administered at a rate of 100 ml/h intravenously. It is important to avoid rapid infusion of large volumes of glucose-containing solutions because maternal hyperglycemia may cause neonatal hypoglycemia immediately after delivery. Thus, if rapid intravenous hydration is necessary before the use of conduction anesthesia, non–glucose-containing solutions should be used. If blood glucose concentration is >120 mg/dl (>6.7 mmol/l), short-acting insulin may be administered via infusion at a rate of 1 U/h intravenously. Adjust the dosage to maintain the blood glucose level within the range of 70–120 mg/dl (3.9–6.7 mmol/l). Insulin infusion should be discontinued immediately before delivery and, in most cases, will not need to be resumed postpartum (Jovanovic 2004).

## OBSTETRIC MANAGEMENT

### FETAL SURVEILLANCE

Use of fetal ultrasound for detection of congenital anomalies is suggested for women with GDM who are suspected of having preexisting diabetes (A1C values >6.5%, fasting plasma glucose levels >125 mg/dl [≥7.0 mmol/l], or random glucose >200 mg/dl [11.1 mmol/l] at first visit), because of the increased risk of major congenital malformations. Use of ultrasound measurements to detect fetal macrosomia as a guide to GDM treatment is considered in the section on metabolic goals and surveillance. Decisions regarding the commencement and frequency of surveillance for fetal well-being should be influenced by the severity of maternal hyperglycemia and the presence of other adverse clinical factors, such as past poor obstetrical history or coincident hypertensive disorders. At a minimum, mothers with GDM should be taught to monitor fetal movements during the last 8–10 weeks of pregnancy and to report immediately any reduction in the perception of fetal movements. Data are not available to demonstrate the optimal application of biophysical fetal monitoring, or which method is superior: nonstress testing, contraction stress testing, or biophysical profile. The ACOG (2001) has suggested that a reasonable approach would be to manage patients with gestational diabetes who require insulin, whose GDM is not well controlled, or who have other risk factors such as a poor obstetric history or hypertension, the same as individuals with preexisting diabetes. It is recognized that no fetal surveillance method is always able to detect fetal compromise. Data are insufficient to determine whether surveillance beyond self-monitoring of fetal movements is indicated in women with GDM continuing to meet the targets of glycemic control with MNT/physical activity regimens and in whom fetal growth is appropriate for gestational age. The rate of intervention is low for such well-controlled GDM pregnancies. As more women are diagnosed with milder gestational diabetes under the new diagnostic recommendations, it will be particularly important to determine the most efficient and cost-effective approach to determining fetal well-being.

## MATERNAL SURVEILLANCE

The frequency of spontaneous preterm birth may be increased in women with untreated GDM (Yogev 2007). Use of corticosteroids to enhance fetal lung maturity should not be withheld because of a diagnosis of GDM, but intensified monitoring of maternal glucose levels is indicated, and a temporary addition or increase of insulin doses may be necessary. The risk of hypertensive disorders also is increased in women with GDM. Studies of nondiabetic women with gestational hypertension suggest that treatment is not indicated during pregnancy in the absence of albuminuria or other signs of target organ damage, but studies of gestational hypertension in women with GDM are not available. Measurement of blood pressure and urinary protein is recommended at each prenatal visit to detect the development of preeclampsia, for which standard treatment methods should be applied in women with GDM.

Assessment of maternal capillary glucose during labor is recommended to prevent maternal hyperglycemia and fetal hypoxia and neonatal hypoglycemia. Prospective studies are needed to determine the frequency of measurement and the optimal glucose levels that are associated with the best perinatal outcome.

Discussion of timing and route of delivery in gestational diabetes is beyond the scope of this monograph. The reader is referred to a recent consensus publication sponsored jointly by the NICHD and the SMFM, which outlines recommendations for timing of delivery in various high-risk situations (Spong 2011). A recent statewide population-based study suggested that the risk of infant death after delivery at 39 completed weeks or 40 completed weeks is lower than the risk of stillbirth associated with another week *in utero* (Rosenstein 2012). Thus, a policy of delivery between 39 and 40 weeks appears appropriate for patients with well-controlled gestational diabetes.

## SELECTED READINGS

Academy of Nutrition and Dietetics (formerly American Dietetic Association): *Medical Nutrition Therapy, Evidence-Based Guides for Practice: Gestational Diabetes Mellitus Evidence-Based Guide for Practice*. Chicago, IL, American Dietetic Association, 2008

American Diabetes Association: *The Official Pocket Guide to Diabetic Exchanges*. Alexandria, VA, American Diabetes Association, 2011

American Diabetes Association and American Dietetic Association: *Choose Your Foods: Plan Your Meals, a guide to planning meals for diabetes*. Alexandria, VA, American Diabetes Association, 2009

American Diabetes Association: Gestational diabetes mellitus (Position Statement). *Diabetes Care* 27 (Suppl. 1):S88–S90, 2004

Crowther CA, Hiller JE, Moss JR, McPhee AJ, Jeffries WJ, Robinson JS, for the Australian Carbohydrate Intolerance Study in Pregnant Women (ACHOIS) Trial Group: Effect of treatment of gestational diabetes mellitus on pregnancy outcomes. *N Engl J Med* 352:2477–2486, 2005

Diabetes Care and Education Practice Group, American Dietetic Association: Diabetes and pregnancy. *On The Cutting Edge* 28:9–17, 2007

Hyperglycemia and Adverse Pregnancy Outcome Study Cooperative Research Group: Hyperglycemia and adverse pregnancy outcomes. *N Engl J Med* 358:1991–2002, 2008

Institute of Medicine, National Research Council: *Weight Gain During Pregnancy: Reexamining the Guidelines*. Rasmussen KM, Yaktine AL, Eds. Washington, DC, National Academies Press, 2009

Institute of Medicine, Food and Nutrition Board: *Dietary Reference Intakes: The Essential Guide to Nutrient Requirements*. Washington, DC, National Academies Press, 2006

Landon MB, Spong CY, Thom E, et al., for the Eunice Kennedy Shriver National Institute of Child Health and Human Development Maternal-Fetal Medicine Units Network: A multicenter randomized trial of treatment for mild gestational diabetes. *N Engl J Med* 361:1339–1348, 2009

Metzger BE, Gabbe SG, Persson B, et al.; for the IADPSG: International Association of Diabetes and Pregnancy St,dy Groups recommendations on the diagnosis and classification of hyperglycemia in pregnancy. *Diab Care* 22:676–682, 2010

Ratner RE, Christophi CA, Metzger BE, et al.: Prevention of diabetes in women with a history of GDM: effects of metformin and lifestyle interventions. *JCEM* 93:4774–4779, 2008

# REFERENCES

Academy of Nutrition and Dietetics (formerly American Dietetic Association): *Medical Nutrition Therapy, Evidence-Based Guides for Practice: Gestational Diabetes Mellitus Evidence-Based Guide for Practice.* Chicago, IL, American Dietetic Association, 2008

American College of Obstetricians and Gynecologists: Exercise during pregnancy and the postpartum period. ACOG Committee Opinion No. 267. *Obstet Gynecol* 99:171–173, 2002 (reaffirmed 2009)

American College of Obstetricians and Gynecologists: Gestational diabetes. ACOG Practice Bulletin No. 30. *Obstet Gynecol* 98:525–538, 2001 (reaffirmed 2010)

American Diabetes Association: Standards of medical care in diabetes—2013. *Diabetes Care* 36 (Suppl. 1):S11–S66, 2013

American Diabetes Association: Standards of medical care in diabetes—2011. *Diabetes Care* 34 (Suppl. 1):S11–S61, 2011

Artal R, Romen Y, Wiswell R: Fetal bradycardia induced by maternal exercise. *Lancet* 2:258–260, 1984

Buchanan TA, Kjos SL, Schafer U, et al.: Utility of fetal measurements in the management of gestational diabetes mellitus. *Diabetes Care* 21 (Suppl. 2):B99–B106, 1998

Carpenter MW, Sady SP, Hoegsberg B, Sady MA, Haydon B, Cullinane EM, Coustan DR, Thompson PD: Fetal heart rate response to maternal exertion. *JAMA* 259: 3006–3009, 1988

Chan LY, Yeung JH, Lau TK: Placental transfer of rosiglitazone in the first trimester of human pregnancy. *Fertil Steril* 83:955–958, 2005

Collings C, Curet LB: Fetal heart rate response to maternal exercise. *Am J Obstet Gynecol* 151:498–501, 1985

Crowther CA, Hiller JE, Moss JR, McPhee AJ, Jeffries WJ, Robinson JS, for the Australian Carbohydrate Intolerance Study in Pregnant Women (ACHOIS) Trial Group: Effect of treatment of gestational diabetes mellitus on pregnancy outcomes. *N Engl J Med* 352:2477–2486, 2005

de Veciana M, Major CA, Morgan MA, Asrat T, Toohey JS, Lien JM, Evans AT: Postprandial versus preprandial blood glucose monitoring in women with gestational diabetes mellitus requiring insulin therapy. *N Engl J Med* 333:1237–1241, 1995

de Veciana M, Trail PA, Evans AT, Dulaney K: A comparison of oral acarbose and insulin in women with gestational diabetes. *Obstet Gynecol* 99 (Suppl.):5S, 2002

Diabetes Care and Education Practice Group, American Dietetic Association: Diabetes and pregnancy. *On the Cutting Edge* 28:9–17, 2007

Dornhorst A, Nicholls JSD, Probst F, Paterson CM, Hollier KL, Elkeles RS, Beard RW: Calorie restriction for treatment of gestational diabetes. *Diabetes* 40 (Suppl. 2):S161–S164, 1991

Durak EP, Jovanovic-Peterson L, Peterson CM: Comparative evaluation of uterine response to exercise on five aerobic machines. *Am J Obstet Gynecol* 162:754–756, 1990

Dye TD, Knox KL, Artal R, Aubry RH, Wojtowycz MA: Physical activity, obesity, and diabetes in pregnancy. *Am J Epidemiol* 146:961–965, 1997

Elliott BD, Langer O, Schenker S, Johnson RF: Insignificant transfer of glyburide occurs across the human placenta. *Am J Obstet Gynecol* 165:807–812, 1991

Freinkel N, Metzger BE, Phelps RL, Dooley SC, Ogata ES, Radvany RM, Belton A: Gestational diabetes mellitus: heterogeneity of maternal age, weight, insulin secretion, HLA antigens, and islet cell antibodies and the impact of maternal metabolism on pancreatic b-cell somatic development in the offspring. *Diabetes* 34 (Suppl. 2):1–7, 1985

HAPO Study Cooperative Research Group: Hyperglycemia and adverse pregnancy outcomes. *N Engl J Med* 358:1991–2002, 2008

Hebert MF, Ma X, Naraharisetti SB, Krudys KM, et al.: Are we optimizing gestational diabetes treatment with glyburide?: The pharmacologic basis for better clinical practice. *Clin Pharmacol Ther* 85:607–614, 2009

Hiles RA, Bawdon RE, Petrella EM: Ex vivo human placental transfer of the peptides pramlintide and exentide. *Hum Exp Toxicol* 22:623–628, 2003

Institute of Medicine, National Research Council: *Weight Gain During Pregnancy: Reexamining the Guidelines*. Rasmussen KM, Yaktine AL, Eds. Washington, DC, National Academies Press, 2009

Institute of Medicine, Food and Nutrition Board: *Dietary Reference Intakes: The Essential Guide to Nutrient Requirements*. Washington, DC, National Academies Press, 2006

Jovanovic L: Glucose and insulin requirements during labor and delivery: the case for normoglycemia in pregnancies complicated by diabetes. *Endocr Pract* 10:40–45, 2004

Jovanovic L, Kessler A, Peterson CM: Human maternal and fetal response to graded exercise. *J Appl Physiol* 58:1719–1722, 1985

Jovanovic L, Savas H, Mehta M, et al.: Frequent monitoring of A1c during pregnancy as a treatment tool to guide therapy. *Diabetes Care* 34:53–54, 2010

Jovanovic-Peterson L, Durak EP, Peterson CM: Randomized trial of diet versus diet plus cardiovascular conditioning on glucose levels in gestational diabetes. *Am J Obstet Gynecol* 161:415–419, 1989

Kjos SL, Schaefer-Graf U, Sardesi S, et al.: A randomized controlled trial using glycemic plus fetal ultrasound parameters versus glycemic parameters to determine insulin therapy in gestational diabetes with fasting hyperglycemia. *Diabetes Care* 24:1904–1910, 2001

Knopp RH, Magee MS, Raisys V, Benedetti T: Metabolic effects of hypocaloric diets in management of gestational diabetes. *Diabetes* 40 (Suppl. 2):S165–S171, 1991

Landon MB, Spong CY, Thom E, et al., for the Eunice Kennedy Shriver National Institute of Child Health and Human Development Maternal-Fetal Medicine Units Network: A multicenter randomized trial of treatment for mild gestational diabetes. *N Engl J Med* 361:1339–1348, 2009

Langer O, Rodriguez DA, Xenakis EMJ, McFarland MB, Berkus MD, Arredondo F: Intensified versus conventional management of gestational diabetes. *Am J Obstet Gynecol* 170:1036–1047, 1994

Major CA, Henry MJ, De Veciana M, Morgan MA: The effects of carbohydrate restriction in patients with diet-controlled gestational diabetes. *Obstet Gynecol* 91:600–604, 1998

Mendez-Figueroa H, Daley J, Lopes VV, Coustan DR: Comparing daily versus less frequent blood glucose monitoring in patients with mild gestational diabetes. *J Matern Fetal Neonatal Med* 2013 Mar 21, [Epub ahead of print]

Metzger BE: Summary and recommendations of the Fifth International Workshop-Conference on Gestational Diabetes Mellitus. *Diabetes Care* 30 (Suppl. 2):S197–S201, 1991

Metzger BE, Buchanan TA, Coustan DR, et al.: Summary and Recommendations of the Fifth International Workshop-Conference on Gestational Diabetes Mellitus. *Diabetes Care* 30(Suppl. 2):S251–S260, 2007

Metzger BE, Gabbe SG, Persson B, et al., for the IADPSG: International Association of Diabetes and Pregnancy Study Groups recommendations on the diagnosis and classification of hyperglycemia in pregnancy. *Diabetes Care* 22:676–682, 2010

Omori Y, Jovanovic L: Proposal for the reconsideration of the definition of gestational diabetes mellitus. *Diabetes Care* 28:1592–1593, 2005

O'Sullivan JB, Mahan CM: Criteria for the oral glucose tolerance test in pregnancy. *Diabetes* 13:278–285, 1964

Parretti E, Meccaci F, Papini M, Cioni R, Carignani L, Mignosa M, La Torre P, Mello G: Third-trimester maternal blood glucose levels from diurnal profiles in nondiabetic pregnancies: correlation with sonographic parameters of fetal growth. *Diabetes Care* 24:1319–1323, 2001

Pederson O, Beck-Nielsen H, Heding L: Increased insulin receptors after exercise in patients with insulin-dependent diabetes mellitus. *N Engl J Med* 302:886–892, 1980

Peterson CM, Jovanovic-Peterson L: Percentage of carbohydrate and glycemic response to breakfast, lunch, and dinner in women with gestational diabetes. *Diabetes* 40 (Suppl. 2):172–174, 1991

Pollex EK, Feig DS, Lubetsky A, Yip PM, Koren G: Insulin glargine safety in pregnancy: a transplacental transfer study. *Diabetes Care* 33:29–33, 2010

Pomerance JJ, Gluck L, Lynch VA: Maternal exercise as a screening test for utero-placental insufficiency. *Obstet Gynecol* 44:383–387, 1974

Ratner RE, Christophi CA, Metzger BE, et al.: Prevention of diabetes in women with a history of GDM: effects of metformin and lifestyle interventions. *JCEM* 93:4774–4779, 2008

Reader DM: Medical nutrition therapy and lifestyle interventions. *Diabetes Care* 30 (Suppl. 2):S188–S193, 2007

Reader D, Splett P, Gunderson EP, for the Diabetes Care and Education Dietetic Practice Group: Impact of gestational diabetes mellitus nutrition practice guidelines implemented by registered dietitians on pregnancy outcomes. *J Am Diet Assoc* 106:1426–1433, 2006

Rizzo T, Metzger BE, Burns WJ, Burns K: Correlations between antepartum maternal metabolism and intelligence of offspring. *N Engl J Med* 325:911–916, 1991

Rosenstein MG, Cheng YW, Snowden JM, et al.: The risk of stillbirth and infant death stratified by gestational age in women with GDM. *Am J Obstet Gynecol* 206:309.e1–e7, 2012

Rowan JA, et al., for the MiG Trial Investigators: Metformin versus insulin for the treatment of gestational diabetes. *N Engl J Med* 358:2003–2015, 2008

Sacks DA, Hadden DR, Maresh M, et al., for the HAPO Study Cooperative Research Group: Frequency of gestational diabetes mellitus at collaborating centers based on IADPSG consensus panel-recommended criteria. *Diabetes Care* 35:526–528, 2012

Silverman BL, Rizzo T, Green OC, Cho NH, Winter RJ, Ogata ES, Richards GE, Metzger BE: Long-term prospective evaluation of offspring of diabetic mothers. *Diabetes* 40 (Suppl. 2):S121–S125, 1991

Spong CY, Mercer BM, D'Alton M, et al.: Timing of indicated late-preterm and early-term birth, NICHD/SMFM consensus. *Obstet Gynecol* 118:323–333, 2011

Vanky E, Stridsklev S, Heimstad R, et al.: Metformin versus placebo from first trimester to delivery in polycystic ovary syndrome: a randomized, controlled multicenter study. *J Clin Endocrinol Metab* 95:E448–E455, 2010

Vanky E, Zahlsen K, Spigset O, Carlsen SM: Placental passage of metformin in women with polycystic ovary syndrome. *Fertil Steril* 83:1575–1578, 2005

World Health Organization: Diabetes Programme: About diabetes. Available at http://www.who.int/diabetes/action_online/basics/en/index1.html. Accessed 27 September 2012

Yogev Y, Langer O: Spontaneous delivery and gestational diabetes: the impact of glycemic control. *Arch Gynecol Obstet* 276:361–365, 2007

Zárate A, Ochoa R, Hernández M, Basurto L: Eficacia de la acarbose para controlar el deterioro de la tolerancia a la glucose durante la gestación. *Ginecol Obstet Mex* 68:42–45, 2000

# Neonatal Care of Infants of Mothers with Diabetes

# Highlights
## Neonatal Care of Infants of Mothers with Diabetes

■ Although many infants of mothers with diabetes (IDMs) have an uneventful perinatal course, there is still an increased rate of complications.

■ Of factors influencing neonatal morbidity in diabetic pregnancies, the most significant single factor is the gestational age of the pregnancy.

■ Maintenance of a normal metabolic state, including euglycemia, should diminish but will not eradicate the increased potential for perinatal and neonatal morbidities.

■ IDMs optimally should be delivered in tertiary care centers with specialized management.

■ Resuscitation requires a fully equipped area and knowledgeable personnel. Evaluation of the IDM should include observation for macrosomia, birth injury, avoidance of asphyxia, presence of congenital malformations, respiratory distress, and hypoglycemia.

■ Nursery care of the infant can be accomplished in a regular nursery or special-care unit if one exists in the delivery hospital. The more appropriate the weight relative to the gestational age of the infant, the greater chance for care in a regular nursery.

# Neonatal Care of Infants of Mothers with Diabetes

The infant of the mother with diabetes (IDM) is an excellent example of the morbidities that may exist in the neonate because of maternal disease (Cowett 1991b). Developmentally, the normal neonate is in a transitional state of glucose homeostasis. The fetus is completely dependent on his or her mother for glucose transfer in utero, and maintenance of glucose homeostasis may be a significant problem. The neonate must maintain a balance between glucose deficiency and excess. The dependence of the conceptus on the mother for continuous substrate delivery contrasts with the variable and intermittent exogenous oral intake by the neonate. Development of homeostasis results from a balance between substrate availability and developmental hormonal, sympathomimetic, and enzymatic systems (Cowett 1991c). The precarious nature of this balance is reinforced by the numerous morbidities producing or associated with altered states of neonatal glucose homeostasis.

Although many IDMs have an uneventful perinatal course, there is still an increased risk of complications, even in the infant born to a woman with gestational diabetes. This section highlights specific factors that are important in the immediate care of the IDM in the delivery room, in the nursery, and subsequently after discharge from the hospital. The IDM has been the subject of extensive reviews (Cowett 1988c, 1991b, 1991c; Lee 2006; Toker-Maimon 2006; Yang 2006).

## PERINATAL MORTALITY AND MORBIDITY

The physician responsible for the care and delivery of the mother should inform the physician responsible for the care of the neonate well in advance of delivery. Factors of importance include the following:

- Knowledge of the character of the maternal diabetes (including diabetes type and degree of glucose and blood pressure control)
- Prior pregnancy history
- Complications occurring during the pregnancy (including results of fetal monitoring for evaluation of fetal size and maturity, episodes of maternal infection, vaginal bleeding, and medications administered)

Knowing these facts allows the physician caring for the neonate to anticipate many of the potential fetal and neonatal complications. These factors determine whether a pediatric provider or neonatologist needs to be present at delivery, although in many institutions delivery of a mother with diabetes always will have pediatric personnel in attendance.

Although some have concluded that peripheral hospitals away from a centralized facility should offer to manage pregnant women with type 1 diabetes (T1D) only if they have an antenatal or endocrine unit and a neonatal intensive care unit (Traub 1987, Cowett 1991a), all pregnant women with diabetes may not be able to be transferred to a centralized facility for care. The physicians caring for the mother and for the neonate, however, must foresee any complications that may arise.

Hanson (1986) evaluated factors influencing neonatal morbidity in diabetic pregnancies. In 92 consecutive pregnancies, those with severe morbidity had the following:

- Longer duration of maternal diabetes
- Shorter gestational age at birth
- Higher rates of cesarean section
- Higher frequency of preeclampsia

The most significant single factor was the gestational age of the pregnancy. Glucose control between 70 and 153 mg/dl (3.8 and 8.5 mmol/l) did not influence morbidity. Thus, the maintenance of a normal metabolic state including euglycemia should diminish, but will not completely eradicate, the increased perinatal and neonatal mortality and morbidities of diabetic pregnancy.

The role of maternal hyperglycemia and the impact on neonatal outcome has been reported (Stenhouse 2006). The authors showed that neonates were ~48 g heavier at birth for each 18 mg/dl increase in maternal glycemia in 4,681 pregnancies. With the increase in birth weight, there also was an increased risk of complications in the neonatal period. Maternal diabetes still remains as the major independent risk factor for fetal macrosomia. Rates of congenital anomalies are still 2–5 times higher in the IDM than the rates in infants born to nondiabetic women, and these rates have not changed over the past 20 years (Wyatt 2004). Thus, the neonatologist must be aware that the newborn of a woman with diabetes should be treated as high-risk until proven otherwise.

## RESUSCITATION

As with any neonate who is considered high-risk, immediately after delivery, the IDM requiring resuscitation and stabilization should be taken care of in a designated resuscitation area. As noted by the *Guidelines for Perinatal Care* (Lockwood 2007), resuscitation should be carried out in a fully equipped area illuminated to at least 100 foot-candles and containing equipment required for skilled resuscitation (Table 10.1). A more detailed accounting can be obtained from the guidelines (Lockwood 2007). Likewise, specific personnel should be available, dedicated to devoting their complete attention to the neonate. The American Heart Association and American Academy of Pediatrics have produced materials to teach resuscitation skills (Lockwood 2007, American Academy of Pediatrics 2011). All neonates need to be dried off initially to maintain as close to a neutral thermal environment as possible. Evaluation of the IDM in the resuscitation room requires observation for multiple factors (Tables 10.1 and 10.2).

## Table 10.1 Equipment Required in Resuscitation

- An overhead source of radiant heat that can be regulated relative to the neonate's body temperature
- Table with equipment (devices to provide positive pressure ventilation, laryngoscope, endotracheal tube, etc.)
- Oxygen, compressed air, and suction dedicated to the neonate
- Trays with medications, fluids (epinephrine, normal saline)
- Wall clock
- Charting surface
- Catheters, needles, stopcocks, infusion pumps

## Table 10.2 Required Observation Checklist for Infants of Mothers with Diabetes in the Resuscitation Room

- Poor respiratory effort
- Birth injury
- Congenital malformations
- Erythremia
- Evidence of macrosomia
- Respiratory distress

## MACROSOMIA, BIRTH INJURY, AND ASPHYXIA

The neonate of the woman with poorly controlled diabetes often will appear macrosomic (>4 kg [>8 lb, 13 oz] at term or >90th percentile in weight for gestational age [American College of Obstetricians and Gynecologists 2005]) in contrast to neonates born to the mother with well-controlled diabetes and the nondiabetic nonobese mother (Cowett 1991b). A consequence of undetected fetal macrosomia may be a difficult vaginal delivery because of shoulder dystocia with resultant birth injury or asphyxia (Table 10.3).

Injury to the brachial plexus may appear with a variety of presentations because the nerves of the brachial plexus may be damaged. In addition to the obvious injury to the nerves of the arm, diaphragmatic paralysis occurs if the phrenic nerve is affected. Because of the associated organomegaly in the IDM, hemorrhage in the abdominal organs is possible, specifically in the liver and adrenal glands. Hemorrhage in the external genitalia of these large neonates has been noted.

Because the neonates are at high risk, intrapartum monitoring is helpful to minimize potential complications. At delivery, the nursing personnel evaluating

## Table 10.3 Potential Birth Injuries in Infants of Mothers with Diabetes

- Brachial plexus injury
- External genitalia hemorrhage
- Abdominal organ injury
- Facial palsy
- Cephalohematoma
- Ocular hemorrhage
- Clavicular fracture
- Subdural hemorrhage
- Diaphragmatic paralysis

the neonate assign Apgar scores at 1 and 5 min to document the adequacy of transition from in utero to extrauterine existence. Although there are many reasons for poor transition among IDMs, relative macrosomia may predispose the fetus and newborn to fetal acidemia. Thus, a cord pH provides an easily obtainable early biochemical assessment of the fetus.

Asphyxia may complicate diabetic deliveries and can result in multiorgan dysfunction. It may affect respiratory, renal, and central nervous system (CNS) functions acutely but also may result in hematological (thrombocytopenia, disseminated intravascular coagulation), metabolic (syndrome of inappropriate antidiuretic hormone secretion, hypocalcemia), myocardial, and hepatic abnormalities. Stabilization of altered hemodynamics (hypotension, poor perfusion, acidemia) is a priority followed by decreased fluid intake because of the potential of renal and CNS injury.

## CONGENITAL ANOMALIES

Although most of the morbidity and mortality data for the IDM have shown improvement with advances in the care of the mothers during pregnancy, congenital anomalies remain a major unresolved problem. The two- to fivefold increase in the incidence of congenital anomalies in the IDM has been long noted in most centers and remains a frequent contributor to perinatal mortality (Miller 1981, Ballard 1984, Goldman 1986, Schwartz 2000, Wren 2003, Touger 2005, Hay 2012; Table 10.4).

## Table 10.4 Discrete Patterns of Congenital Malformations in Infants of Mothers with Diabetes

- Major congenital heart disease
- Musculoskeletal deformities, including caudal regression syndrome
- CNS deformities (anencephaly, spina bifida, hydrocephalus)

The prevalence and spectrum of cardiovascular malformations in infants born to mothers with preexisting diabetes compared with that in infants of nondiabetic mothers has been assessed prospectively in a geographic region of the U.K. between 1995 and 2000 (Wren 2003). There were 192,618 live births; cardiovascular malformations occurred in 3.6% of infants of diabetic pregnancies and in 0.74% of infants of nondiabetic pregnancies (odds ratio 5.0, 95% confidence interval 3.3 to 7.8). There was a more than threefold increase in transposition of the great vessels, truncus arteriosus, and tricuspid atresia among infants born to mothers with diabetes.

The pathogenesis of the increased frequency of congenital anomalies among the IDMs remains obscure (Touger 2005). Several etiologies have been proposed to account for the incidence of anomalies:

- Hyperglycemia, either preconceptional or postconceptional
- Hypoglycemia
- Uteroplacental vascular disease
- Genetic predisposition

Although there are data to support each proposal, the evidence is best for the preconceptional and early postconceptional hyperglycemia etiology (Kitzmiller 1978, Miller 1981, Fuhrmann 1983, Ballard 1984, Goldman 1986, Freinkel 1990, Metzger 1990). The preponderance of evidence indicates that early rigid glucose control will minimize the incidence of anomalies (Schwartz 2000). The critical period of teratogenesis occurs before the seventh week postconception. In contrast, poor glucose control later in pregnancy carries a higher risk of macrosomia, intrauterine growth restriction, asphyxia, and fetal death (Hay 2012).

Cardiomyopathy in the IDM can be congestive or hypertrophic. Hypertrophic cardiomyopathy in neonates has been associated with poorly controlled diabetes in the mother and neonatal hypoglycemia. Respiratory distress can be accompanied by septal hypertrophy (Way 1979, Reeler 1988), with resolution of symptoms within 2–4 weeks and of the hypertrophy within 2–12 months (Mace 1979). Hypertrophy of the interventricular septum and walls of the right and left ventricles also has been documented (Breitweser 1980). Profound hypoglycemia after birth, consistent with the metabolic effects of neonatal hyperinsulinism, has been strongly associated with septal hypertrophy (Ballard 1984). Fetal hyperinsulinism may contribute directly to septal hypertrophy.

Although cardiac hypertrophy, apart from congenital heart disease, has been recognized in autopsies of IDMs for the past three decades, it is now understood that some IDMs have a peculiar form of subaortic stenosis similar to the idiopathic hypertrophic subaortic stenosis found in adults (Halliday 1981). This particular entity may be associated with symptomatic congestive heart failure. As with the adult variant, in these neonates, therapy with digoxin is contraindicated because the resultant increased myocardial contractility has been reported to be deleterious. Propranolol appears to be the therapeutic drug of choice. Clinically, this disorder resolves spontaneously over a period of weeks to months with correction of the echocardiographic features as well.

## RESPIRATORY DISTRESS

Respiratory distress, including respiratory distress syndrome (RDS), is a frequent and potentially severe complication in the IDM, although the trend toward delivering patients with diabetes later rather than earlier in gestation (assisted by improvement in the assessment of fetal well-being) is lowering the incidence. Neonatal RDS (pathological correlate: hyaline membrane disease) develops because of lung immaturity in the neonate and remains a major cause of mortality. The relative risk of RDS in the IDM ≤38 weeks gestational age was once reported to be more than five times higher than in neonates of nondiabetic mothers (Robert 1976). Other causes of respiratory distress in the IDM exist as well (Table 10.5).

### Table 10.5. Causes of Respiratory Distress in Infants of Mothers with Diabetes, Other Than Respiratory Distress Syndrome

- Cardiac disease
- Pneumomediastinum
- Diaphragmatic hernia
- Pneumothorax
- Meconium aspiration
- Transient tachypnea

RDS has a typical course that is manifested by increasing oxygen requirements due to progressive respiratory compromise. Tachypnea, intercostal and subcostal retractions, nasal flaring, and expiratory grunting appearing in the first few minutes to hours of life are the cardinal signs of the disease. In uncomplicated cases, the disease usually peaks by 72 h of age. With the use of exogenous surfactant, the time course of RDS has been greatly shortened for the majority of infants. Complications commonly associated with RDS include air leaks (the latter has been reduced by surfactant), the presence of a persistent patent ductus arteriosus in preterm infants, and bronchopulmonary dysplasia in preterm infants requiring prolonged ventilatory support and high ambient oxygen concentrations. Both of these conditions may significantly lengthen the clinical course of an otherwise self-limited disease. RDS should be managed with particular attention to the following:

- Fluid administration and avoiding unneeded volume expansion
- Supplemental oxygen
- Continuous positive airway pressure
- Ventilator support when necessary
- Exogenous surfactant if intubation is needed

To date, there have been no controlled trials of administration of exogenous surfactant to IDMs who were delivered with RDS. This therapy is being utilized clinically for treatment of RDS in the premature IDM in many centers around the U.S.

## HYPOGLYCEMIA

A rapid decrease in plasma glucose concentration after delivery is characteristic of the IDM. The blood or plasma glucose concentration that is thought to be abnormal continues to be debated among newborn providers (Adamkin 2011). For many practitioners, however, values <35 mg/dl (<1.9 mmol/l) at term are considered abnormal and may occur within 30 min after clamping the umbilical vessels (Srinivasan 1986). Factors that influence the degree of hypoglycemia include previous maternal glucose homeostasis and maternal glycemia during delivery (Cowett 1991c). A mother whose diabetes has been controlled inadequately during pregnancy will have stimulated the fetal pancreas to synthesize excessive insulin, which may be readily released. Administration of intravenous dextrose during the intrapartum period, which results in maternal hyperglycemia >125 mg/dl (>6.9 mmol/l), will be reflected in the fetus and will exaggerate the neonate's normal postdelivery fall in plasma glucose concentration. Hypoglycemia may persist for 48 h or may develop after 24 h (Lin 1989).

The neonate exhibits transitional control of glucose metabolism, which suggests that a multiplicity of factors affect homeostasis. Many of the factors are similar to those that influence homeostasis in the adult. There is blunted splanchnic (hepatic) responsiveness to insulin in both the preterm and term neonate, however, compared with the adult (Cowett 1988b). What has not been studied in the IDM are the many counterinsulin hormones that influence metabolism (Cowett 1988a, 1988b; Lin 1989). If insulin is the primary glucoregulatory hormone, then counterinsulin hormones assist in balancing the effect of insulin and other factors.

## NURSERY CARE

The presence of the specific morbidities discussed thus far requires specialized care by individuals who have the knowledge, training, and experience to handle subsequent care and follow-up. Given this consideration, the clinician should decide whether to observe the IDM in a special-care nursery or follow the neonate in the regular nursery, assuming both exist in the delivering hospital, or transfer the infant to a special-care unit at another health center (Table 10.6). Even if the IDM can be cared for in the regular nursery, specific metabolic abnormalities should be looked for, including the following:

- Hypoglycemia
- Hypocalcemia
- Hypomagnesemia
- Erythremia
- Hyperbilirubinemia

## GLUCOSE HOMEOSTASIS

Relative to glucose metabolism, the IDM is a prime example of the potential of glucose disequilibrium in the neonate. Because of the transitional nature of glucose homeostasis in the newborn period in general, accentuation of disequilib-

**Table 10.6 Factors Indicating That the Infant of a Mother with Diabetes Will Need Care in a Special-Care Nursery**

- Asphyxia
- Birth injury
- Congenital malformations
- History of maternal insulin administration
- Hypoglycemia
- Tetany
- Large or small for gestational age

rium may be enhanced in the IDM, secondary to metabolic alterations in the mother. Preventive therapy should include rigid control of maternal blood glucose levels during pregnancy and delivery.

Similar to infants of nondiabetic pregnancies, IDMs can appear asymptomatic even with a relatively low plasma glucose concentration. This may be due to the initial brain stores of glycogen; other etiologies include the use of alternative substrates for oxidative metabolism because concentrations of lactate and ketone bodies frequently are elevated shortly after birth.

Although a laboratory determination of blood glucose is the most accurate method, it does not provide results in real time, which are needed for screening for hypoglycemia. Bedside reagent test-strip glucose analyzers can be used if the test is performed with proper quality control measures and if providers are aware of the limitations of such devices (Adamkin 2011). In view of the limitations of bedside rapid determinations of blood glucose concentration, abnormal values should be confirmed with stat laboratory testing.

IDMs may require parenteral treatment for maintenance of carbohydrate homeostasis. Early administration of oral feeding shortly after birth may be beneficial to maintain plasma glucose concentrations that are not depressed.

The neonate who has a glucose concentration <40 mg/dl (<2.2 mmol/l) at ≤4 h of age (for both the term and preterm neonate) in the presence of symptoms (see Table 10.7) should be treated with glucose administered intravenously. Bolus injection without subsequent infusion will only exaggerate the hypoglycemia by a rebound mechanism and is contraindicated. Minibolus therapy (200 mg/kg or 2 cc/kg of 10% dextrose) has been demonstrated to avoid the rebound hypoglycemia (Lilien 1980) and can be followed with infusion of 6–8 mg/kg/min of glucose. Once plasma glucose stabilizes to >45 mg/dl (>2.5 mmol/l), the infusion may be slowly decreased while oral feedings are initiated and advanced. If symptomatic hypoglycemia persists, higher glucose rates of ≥8–12 mg/kg min (3.6–5.5 mg/lb min) may be necessary and may necessitate insertion of an umbilical venous catheter to use higher dextrose concentrations and to avoid excessive fluid administration. Because most neonates are asymptomatic, glucagon administration to prevent hypoglycemia after delivery does not appear warranted. Furthermore, glucagon may stimulate insulin release, which may exaggerate the tendency for hypoglycemia.

## Table 10.7 Signs and Symptoms of Neonatal Hypoglycemia

| | | |
|---|---|---|
| Abnormal cry | Convulsions | Jitteriness |
| Apathy | Cyanosis | Lethargy |
| Apnea | Hypothermia | Tremors |
| Cardiac arrest | Hypotonia | Tachypnea |

Prompt recognition and treatment of the hypoglycemic neonate has minimized sequelae. A long-standing area of uncertainty is the potential contribution of hypoglycemia to brain injury. Glucose is the principal substrate for cerebral metabolism and hypoglycemia can cause neuronal and glial injury (Banker 1967, Koivisto 1972). The independent effect of hypoglycemia, however, is difficult to determine in the clinical setting. In prospective evaluations of low–birth weight infants, moderate hypoglycemia (<2.6 mmol/l) has been associated with an increase in neurodevelopmental sequelae (Lucas 1988). Unfortunately, rigorous randomized trials probably cannot be conducted to clarify this issue.

With the use of magnetic resonance imaging (MRI), the effect of hypoglycemia has been investigated in more recent cohorts of infants to determine whether a specific neurologic pattern of injury can be observed in infants who experienced symptomatic neonatal hypoglycemia (Karimzadeh 2011). Ninety percent of infants showed abnormal signal in the posterior cerebral area supporting a hypoglycemia-occipital syndrome. Others have also reported the association between neonatal hypoglycemia and occipital cerebral injury with links to long-term disability, epilepsy, and visual impairment (Filan 2006). Not all reports have confirmed these associations. In a cohort of 35 term infants with symptomatic neonatal hypoglycemia (median glucose level of 1 mmol/l), in the absence of hypoxia-ischemia, patterns of injury on MRI were varied with white matter abnormalities as the most common (94%); a predominant posterior pattern occurred in only 29% (Burns 2008). Twenty-three infants (65%) demonstrated impairments at 18 months that were related to the severity of the white matter injury and not to the location. In spite of this difference, these studies confirm the potential for symptomatic hypoglycemia to be associated with brain injury.

Ultimately, the neonate will require full supplementation orally. Although proprietary formula is available, breast-feeding by the mother is to be encouraged.

## HYPOCALCEMIA AND HYPOMAGNESEMIA

Besides hypoglycemia, hypocalcemia ranks as an important metabolic derangement observed in the IDM (Tsang 1979). During pregnancy, calcium is transferred from mother to fetus concomitant with an increasing hyperparathyroid state in the mother. Calcium concentrations are higher in the fetus than in the mother. This hyperparathyroid state functions as a homeostatic compensation to restore the maternal calcium that is diverted to the fetus. Neither calcitonin nor parathyroid hormone (PTH) crosses the placenta. At birth, serum calcium falls, subsequent to interruption of maternal–fetal calcium transfer. Elevations in PTH and 1,25-dihydroxyvitamin D as early as 24 h of age ensure correction of the low serum calcium concentration.

In a case series of 532 infants born to 332 women with gestational diabetes and 177 women with preexisting T1D, hypoglycemia occurred in 27% of infants and hypocalcemia was documented in only 4% of infants. Low rates of hypocalcemia are speculated to reflect improved blood glucose control during pregnancy and appropriate triage of infants with anticipation of neonatal problems (Cordero 1998).

Hypomagnesemia (<1.5 mg/dl) may occur in IDMs, often in association with hypocalcemia. As with hypocalcemia, the frequency and severity of clinical symptoms are correlated with maternal status. Neonatal magnesium concentration has been correlated with that in the mother as well as with the maternal insulin requirements and concentration of intravenous glucose administered to the neonate (Noguchi 1980). Hypocalcemia in the IDM may be secondary to decreased hypoparathyroid function as a result of the hypomagnesemia. Hypocalcemia and hypomagnesemia may have clinical manifestations similar to those of hypoglycemia in addition to those of tetany and should be treated.

## HYPERBILIRUBINEMIA AND ERYTHREMIA

Hyperbilirubinemia is observed more frequently in the IDM than in the normal neonate. The pathogenesis remains uncertain (Cowett 1988c, 1991b; Yang 2006). Prematurity (biochemical immaturity) has been rejected as an explanation (Burns 2008). Other etiologies of the hyperbilirubinemia have been related to hemolysis with decreased erythrocyte survival. Erythrocyte life span, osmotic fragility, and deformability have not been found to be appreciably different in IDMs who are at risk for hyperbilirubinemia (Taylor 1963, Peevy 1980). Delayed clearance of the bilirubin load, however, measured by pulmonary excretion of carbon monoxide as an index of bilirubin production, may be a factor (Stevenson 1981a, 1981b).

The erythremia (polycythemia is a misnomer, because only the erythrocyte mass is elevated, not the leukocyte count or the platelet count) frequently observed in IDMs may be the most important factor associated with hyperbilirubinemia. Venous hematocrits ≥65–70% have been observed in 20–40% of IDMs during the first days of life, and sometimes have been associated with signs and symptoms of neonatal erythremia, such as jitteriness, seizures, tachypnea, priapism, and oliguria. Therapy with the use of a partial-exchange transfusion (10–15% of total blood volume) through the umbilical vein with plasmanate or 5% albumin has been associated with a rapid resolution of symptoms.

---

## LONG-TERM FOLLOW-UP

What are the long-term effects of maternal diabetes on growth, development, and psychosocial and intellectual capabilities and the risk to the neonate of subsequently developing diabetes?

An early prospective study of growth and development of the IDM suggested that excessive weight is almost 10 times more common in children of mothers with diabetes than unusually low weight, which may represent a potential "return to obesity" noted at birth in this group of neonates (Farquhar 1960). Furthermore, neonates with a birth weight >4 kg (>8 lb, 13 oz) had significant elevations of height or weight at the time of entrance to school (Bibergeil 1975). Vohr (1980) suggested that macrosomia in the IDM may be a predisposing factor for later obesity, because at 7 years of age, 8 of 19 IDMs who had been large for gestational age at birth were obese, whereas only 1 of 14 who had been appropriate for gestational age was obese. When body weight and length and head circumference were evaluated from birth through 48 months of age, children of mothers with poor control during pregnancy showed higher values for weight and the weight-to-height ratio in infancy compared with neonates of well-controlled mothers (Gerlini 1986). Studies have shown that the offspring of a woman with GDM is at increased risk for developing obesity during adolescence and glucose intolerance in young adulthood (Pettitt 1991, Silverman 1991). The development of the metabolic syndrome (obesity, hypertension, dyslipidemia, and glucose intolerance) has been examined among large-for-gestation and appropriate-for-gestation offspring of mothers with or without gestational diabetes at ages 6–11 years of age (Boney 2005). Large-for-gestational-age offspring of mothers with diabetes were at significant risk of developing the metabolic syndrome in childhood (hazard ratio 2.19, 95% confidence interval 1.25–3.82). Furthermore, adult offspring of women with diet-treated gestational diabetes mellitus or T1D are at risk for obesity and the metabolic syndrome (Clausen 2009).

The high frequency of congenital malformations in IDMs may be directly or indirectly associated with neuropsychological handicaps. Cerebral palsy and epilepsy are three to five times higher in IDMs compared with infants of nondiabetic mothers, but the rate of mental retardation is not different (Yssing 1975, Stehbens 1977). When present, the difficulties are related to extremes of maternal age, severity of diabetes, low birth weight for gestational age, or complications during pregnancy. Psychological evaluations of children at 1, 3, and 5 years of age suggested that at 3 and 5 years of age, the IDM is more vulnerable to intellectual impairment, especially if the child was born small for gestational age or if the mother's pregnancy was complicated by ketonuria (Stehbens 1977). This has been confirmed (Rizzo 1991). Data suggest that neurobehavioral development at birth and during childhood may be affected adversely in offspring of women with GDM whose blood glucose levels were less than optimally controlled during the pregnancy (Rizzo 1991). Consistent with these observations are intelligence quotient scores on the Wechsler Intelligence Scale and Bender tests of infants born to mothers with diabetes and gestational diabetes compared with control subjects (Ornoy 2001). Preexisting and gestational diabetes were associated with a lower attention span and motor function of offspring at school age but not their cognitive ability.

The question of whether the IDM has an increased likelihood of developing diabetes is important. If one parent has T1D, it is in the range of 1–6% (Anderson 1981, Kobberling 1986; see also the chapter on prepregnancy counseling). Although family aggregates do exist, transmitted both through and within generations, a simple mode of inheritance is inconsistent with the reported data (Simpson 1970). Some have suggested that a polygenic multifactorial model best explains the reported observations (Anderson 1981). The history of maternal diabetes should not be forgotten.

## SELECTED READINGS

Adamkin DH; Committee on Fetus and Newborn: Postnatal glucose homeostasis in late preterm and term infants. *Pediatrics* 127:575–579, 2011

Hay WW: Care of the infant of the diabetic mother. *Curr Diab Rep* 12:4–15, 2012

## REFERENCES

Adamkin DH, Committee on Fetus and Newborn: Postnatal glucose homeostasis in late preterm and term infants. *Pediatrics* 127:575–579, 2011

American Academy of Pediatrics: *Textbook of Neonatal Resuscitation.* 6th ed. Dallas, TX, American Heart Association, 2011

American Academy of Pediatrics and the American College of Obstetricians and Gynecologists. *Guidelines for Perinatal Care.* 6th ed. Lockwood CJ, Lemmons JA, Eds. Washington, DC, American Academy of Pediatrics, 2007

American College of Obstetricians and Gynecologists Committee on Practice Bulletins: Pregestational diabetes mellitus. ACOG Practice Bulletin No. 60. *Obstet Gynecol* 105:675–685, 2005

Anderson CE, Rotter JI, Rimoin DL: Genetics of diabetes mellitus. In *Diabetes Mellitus.* Vol. 5. Rifkin H, Raskin P, Eds. Bowie, MD, Brady, 1981, p. 79

Ballard J, Holroyde J, Tsang RC, Chan G, Sutherland JM, Knowles HC: High malformation rates and decreased mortality in infants of diabetic mothers managed after the first trimester (1956–1978). *Am J Obstet Gynecol* 148:111–118, 1984

Banker BQ: The neuropathological effects of anoxia and hypoglycemia in the newborn. *Dev Med Child Neurol* 9:544–550, 1967

Bibergeil H, Bodel E, Amendt P: Diabetes and pregnancy: early and late prognoses of children of diabetic mothers. In *Early Diabetes in Early Life.* Carmerini-Davalos RA, Cole HS, Eds. New York, NY, Academic, 1975, p. 427–434

Boney CM, Verma A, Tucker R, Vohr BR, Metabolic syndrome in childhood: association with birth weight, maternal obesity and gestational diabetes mellitus. *Pediatrics* 115:e290–e296, 2005

Breitweser JA, Mayer RA, Sperling MA, Psang RC, Kaplan S: Cardiac septal hypertrophy in hyperinsulinemic infants. *J Pediatr* 96:535–539, 1980

Burns CM, Rutherford MA, Boardman JP, Cowan FM: Patterns of cerebral injury and neurodevelopmental outcomes after symptomatic neonatal hypoglycemia. *Pediatrics* 122:65–74, 2008

Clausen TD, Mathiesen ER, Hansen T, Pedersen O, Jensen DM, Lauenborg J, Schmidt L, Damm P: Overweight and the metabolic syndrome in adult offspring of women with diet-treated gestational diabetes or type 1 diabetes. *J Clin Endocrinol Metab* 94:2464–2470, 2009

Cordero L, Treuer SH, Landon MB, Gabbe SG: Management of infants of diabetic mothers. *Arch Pediatr Adolesc Med* 152:249–254, 1998

Cowett RM.: The infant of the diabetic mother. In *Principles of Perinatal-Neonatal Metabolism*. Cowett RM, Ed. New York, NY, Springer-Verlag, 1991a, p. 278–298

Cowett RM: The infant of the diabetic mother. In *Medical and Surgical Complications of Pregnancy: Effects on the Fetus and Newborn*. Sweet AY, Brown E, Eds. Chicago, IL, Year Book, 1991b, p. 302–319

Cowett RM: Neonatal glucose metabolism. In *Principles of Perinatal-Neonatal Metabolism*. Cowett RM, Ed. New York, NY, Springer-Verlag, 1991c, p. 356–389

Cowett RM: Alpha adrenergic agonists stimulate neonatal glucose production less than beta adrenergic agonists in the lamb. *Metabolism* 37:831–36, 1988a

Cowett RM: Decreased response to catecholamines in the newborn: effect on glucose kinetics in the lamb. *Metabolism* 37:736–740, 1988b

Cowett RM: The metabolic sequelae in the infant of the diabetic mother. In *Endocrinology and Metabolism*. Cohen MP, Foa PP, Eds. *Controversies in Diabetes and Pregnancy*. Jovanovic L, sect. Ed. New York, NY, Springer-Verlag, 1988c, p. 149–171

Farquhar JW: Prognosis for babies born to diabetic mothers in Edinburgh. *Arch Dis Child* 44:36–47, 1960

Filan PM, Inder TE, Cameron FJ, Kean MJ, Hunt RW: Neonatal hypoglycemia and occipital cerebral injury. *J Pediatrics* 148:552–555, 2006

Freinkel N, Ogata E, Metzger BE: The offspring of the mother with diabetes. In *Ellenberg and Rifkin's Diabetes Mellitus: Theory and Practice*. 4th ed. Rifkin H, Porte D Jr., Eds. New York, NY, Elsevier, 1990, p. 651

Fuhrmann K, Reiher H, Semmler K, Fischer M, Glockner E: Prevention of congenital malformations in infants of insulin dependent diabetic mothers. *Diabetes Care* 6:219–223, 1983

Gerlini G, Arachi S, Gori MG, Gloria F, Bonci E, Pachi A, Zuccarini O, Fiore R, Fallucca F: Developmental aspects of the offspring of diabetic mothers. *Acta Endocrinol Suppl* 277:150–155, 1986

Goldman JA, Dicker D, Feldberg D, Yeshaya A, Samuel N, Karp M: Pregnancy outcome in patients with insulin-dependent diabetes mellitus with preconceptional diabetic control: a comparative study. *Am J Obstet Gynecol* 155:193–197, 1986

Halliday HL: Hypertrophic cardiomyopathy in infants of poorly controlled diabetic mothers. *Arch Dis Child* 56:258–263, 1981

Hanson U, Persson B, Stangenberg M: Factors influencing neonatal morbidity in diabetic pregnancy. *Diabetes Res Clin Pract* 3:71–76, 1986

Hay WW: Care of the infant of the diabetic mother. *Curr Diab Rep* 12:4–15, 2012

Karimzadeh P, Tabarestani S, Ghofrani M: Hypoglycemia-occipital syndrome: a specific neurologic syndrome following neonatal hypoglycemia? *J Child Neurol* 26:152–159, 2011

Kitzmiller JL, Cloherty JP, Younger MD, Tabatabaii A, Rothchild SB, Sosnko I, Epstein F, Singh S, Neff RK: Diabetic pregnancy and perinatal morbidity. *Am J Obstet Gynecol* 131:560–568, 1978

Kobberling J, Tillil H: Risk to family members of becoming diabetic: a study on the genetics of type 1 diabetes. *Pediatr Adolesc Endocrinol* 15:26–38, 1986

Koivisto M, Blanco-Sequeriros M, Krause U: Neonatal symptomatic and asymptomatic hypoglycemia; a follow-up study of 151 children. *Dev Med Child Neurol* 14:603–614, 1972

Lee JK: Newborn resuscitation. *Pediatr Rev* 27:e52–e53, 2006

Lilien LD, Pidles RS, Sainivasan G, Voora S, Yeh TF: Treatment of neonatal hypoglycemia with minibolus and intravenous glucose infusion. *J Pediatr* 97:295–298, 1980

Lin HC, Maguire CA, Oh W, Cowett RM: Accuracy and reliability of glucose reflectance meters in the high risk neonate. *J Pediatr* 115:998–1000, 1989

Lucas A, Morley R, Cole TJ: Adverse neurodevelopmental outcome of moderate neonatal hypoglycemia. *BMJ* 297:1304–1308, 1988

Mace S, Hirschfeld SS, Riggs T, Fanaroff AA, Merkatz IR: Echocardiographic abnormalities in infants of diabetic mothers. *J Pediatr* 95:1013–1019, 1979

Metzger BE, Buchanan TA, Eds.: Diabetes and birth defects: insights from the 1980s, prevention in the 1990s. *Diabetes Spectrum* 3:149–184, 1990

Miller E, Hare JW, Cloherty JP, Dunn PJ, Gleason RE, Soeldner JS, Kitzmiller JL: Elevated maternal hemoglobin A1c in early pregnancy and major congenital anomalies in infants of diabetic mothers. *N Engl J Med* 304:1331–1334, 1981

Noguchi A, Erin M, Tsang RC: Parathyroid hormone in hypocalcemia and normocalcemic infants of diabetic mothers. *J Pediatr* 97:112–114, 1980

Ornoy A, Ratzon N, Greenbaum C, Wolf A, Dulizky M: School age children born to diabetic mothers and to gestational diabetes exhibit a high rate of inattention and fine and gross motor impairment. *J Pediatr Endocrinol Metab* 14 (Suppl. 1):S681–S689, 2001

Peevy KJ, Landaw SA, Gross SA: Hyperbilirubinemia in infants of diabetic mothers. *Pediatrics* 66:417–419, 1980

Pettitt DJ, Bennett PH, Saad MF, Charles MA, Nelson RG, Knowler WC: Abnormal glucose tolerance during pregnancy in Pima Indian women: long-term effects on offspring. *Diabetes* 40 (Suppl. 2):S126–S130, 1991

Reeler MD, Kaplan S: Hypertrophic cardiomyopathy in infants of diabetic mothers: an update. *Am J Perinatol* 4:353–358, 1988

Rizzo T, Metzger BE, Nurns WJ, Burns K: Correlations between antepartum maternal metabolism and intelligence of offspring. *N Engl J Med* 325:911–916, 1991

Robert MD, Neff RK, Hubbell JP, Taeusch HW, Avery ME: Association between maternal diabetes and the respiratory distress syndrome in the newborn. *N Engl J Med* 294:357–360, 1976

Schwartz R, Teramo KA: Effects of diabetic pregnancy on the fetus and newborn. *Semin Perinatology* 24:120–135, 2000

Silverman BL, Rizzo T, Green OC, Cho NH, Winter RJ, Ogata ES, Richards GE, Metzger BE: Long-term prospective evaluation of offspring of diabetic mothers. *Diabetes* 40 (Suppl. 2):S121–S125, 1991

Simpson J: Genetics of diabetes mellitus and anomalies in offspring of diabetic mothers. In *The Diabetic Pregnancy: A Perinatal Perspective.* Merkatz IR, Adam PAJ, Eds. New York, NY, Grune & Stratton, 1970, p. 249–260

Srinivasan G, Pildes RS, Cattamanchi G, Vooru S, Lilien LD: Plasma glucose values in normal neonates: a new look. *J Pediatr* 109:114–117, 1986

Stehbens JA, Baker GL, Kitchell M: Outcome at ages 1, 3, and 5 years of children born to diabetic women. *Am J Obstet Gynecol* 127:408–413, 1977

Stenhouse E, Wright DE, Hattersley AT, Millward BA: Maternal glucose levels influence birthweight and "catch-up" and "catch-down" growth in a large contemporary cohort. *Diabet Med* 234:1207–1212, 2006

Stevenson DK, Ostrander CR, Cohen RS, Johnson JD, Schwartz HC: Pulmonary excretion of carbon monoxide in the human infant as an index of bilirubin production. *Eur J Pediatr* 137:255–259, 1981a

Stevenson DK, Ostrander CR, Hopper AO, Cohen RS, Johnson JD: Pulmonary excretion of carbon monoxide as an index of bilirubin production. IIa. Evidence for possible delayed clearance of bilirubin in infants of diabetic mothers. *J Pediatr* 98:822–824, 1981b

Taylor PM, Wolfson J, Bright NH, Britchard EL, Derinoz MN, Watson DW: Hyperbilirubinemia in infants of diabetic mothers. *Biol Neonate* 5:289–298, 1963

Toker-Maimon O, Joseph LJ, Bromiker R, Schimmel MS: Neonatal cardiopulmonary arrest in the delivery room. *Pediatrics* 118:847–888, 2006

Touger L, Looker HC, Krakoff J, Lindsay RS, Cook V, Knowler WC: Early growth in offspring of diabetic mothers. *Diabetes Care* 28:585–589, 2005

Traub AI, Harley JM, Cooper TK, Maguiness S, Hadden DR: Is centralized hospital care necessary for all insulin-dependent pregnant diabetics? *Br J Obstet Gynaecol* 94:957–962, 1987

Tsang RC, Brown DR, Steinchen JJ: Diabetes and calcium disturbances in infants of diabetic mothers. In *The Diabetic Pregnancy: A Perinatal Perspective*. Merkatz IR, Adam PAJ, Eds. New York, NY, Grune & Stratton, 1979, p. 207–225

Vohr BR, Lipsitt LP, Oh W: Somatic growth of children of diabetic mothers with reference to birth size. *J Pediatr* 97:196–119, 1980

Way GL, Wolfe RR, Eshaghpour E, Bender RL, Jaffe RB, Ruttenberg HD: The natural history of hypertrophic cardiomyopathy in infants of diabetic mothers. *J Pediatr* 95:1020–1025, 1979

Wren C, Birrell G, Hawthorne G: Cardiovascular malformations in infants of diabetic mothers. *Heart* 89:1217–1220, 2003

Wyatt JW, Frias JL, Hoyme HE, Jovanovic L, Kaaja R, Brown F, Garg S, Lee-Parritz A, Seely EW, Kerr L, Mattoo V, Tan M, the IONS Study Group: Congenital anomaly rate in offspring of pre-gestational diabetic women treated with insulin lispro during pregnancy. *Diabet Med* 21:2001–2007, 2004

Yang J, Cummings EA, O'Connell C, Jangaard K: Fetal and neonatal outcomes of diabetic pregnancies. *Obstet Gynecol* 108:644–650, 2006

Yssing M: Long-term prognosis of children born to mothers diabetic when pregnant. In *Early Diabetes in Early Life*. Camerini-Davalos RM, Cole HS, Eds. New York, NY, Academic, 1975, p. 575–586

# Index

# J

jitteriness, 163*t*, 164
Jovanovic, L., 113

# K

karyotyping, 122–123
ketoacidosis. *See* diabetic ketoacidosis
(DKA)
ketone, 18, 59, 139
ketone bodies, 162
ketonemia, 59–60, 69, 96
ketonuria, 59–60, 69, 71–72, 136, 138,
165

# L

labor, 127
labor, preterm, 5*t*
laboratory evaluation, 12*t*
lactate, 162
lactation, 82*t*–83*t*, 91*t*, 98, 114
lactation nutrition management, 94–98
lactogenesis, 98
Lantus, 17
laparoscopy, 34
large for gestational age at birth, 162*t*,
165
laryngoscope, 157*t*
laser photocoagulation, 13
late deceleration, 124
Latina population, 33
lecithin-sphingomyelin ratio, 126
lethargy, 163*t*
level II ultrasound, 121–122
Levemir, 17
levonorgestrel, 32
levonorgestrel-containing intrauterine
system (LNG-IUS), 30, 33*t*
levonorgestrel-releasing intrauterine
device (LNG-IUD), 34*t*–35*t*
lifestyle, 15, 71, 138
lifestyle intervention, 140
linoleic acid, 82*t*
lipid based energy, 107
lipid/lipid level, 31–32, 86
listeria, 93
liver, 157
liver disease, 30

liver enzyme, 72
liver function, 69
liver tumor, 31
liver-produced globulin, 31
long-term disability, 163
long-term follow-up, 164–165
low birth weight, 89–90, 92, 140
low–fasting glucose treatment, 17

# M

macronutrient, 81–85, 91, 96
macrosomia
calorie restriction, 139
diagnostic testing and fetal
surveillance, 120*t*
fetal surveillance, 144
fetal surveillance with
ultrasound, 123
infants of mothers with diabetes
(IDMs), 6*t*, 79–80, 156–158,
165
maternal hyperglycemia, 133–134
metabolic management, 141
mode of delivery, 126–127
macular edema, 13
magnesium, 82*t*, 90, 164
magnesium sulfate, 112, 128
magnetic resonance imaging (MRI),
163
malabsorption, 89
mammary development, 98
*Management of Preexisting Diabetes and
Pregnancy* (Kitzmiller 2008), 80, 87,
90–92
manganese, 82*t*
marital problems, 46
masochistic person, 46
mastitis, 98
maternal
acidosis, 127
age, 122
bonding, 49
capillary blood glucose, 145
complications in diabetic
pregnancy, 5*t*
glucose homeostasis, 161
glucose levels, 84
glycemia, 57, 59, 161